Exercise and Sport
in Diabetes

Diabetes

in Practice

Other titles in the Wiley *Diabetes in Practice* Series

Diabetes in Old Age
Paul Finucane and Alan J. Sinclair (Editors)

Prediction, Prevention and Genetic Counseling in IDDM
Jerry P. Palmer (Editor)

Diabetes and Pregnancy:
An International Approach to Diagnosis and Management
Anne Dornhorst and David R. Hadden (Editors)

Diabetic Complications
Ken M. Shaw (Editor)

Childhood and Adolescent Diabetes
Simon Court and Bill Lamb (Editors)

Hypoglycaemia in Clinical Diabetes
Brian M. Frier and B. Miles Fisher (Editors)

Exercise and Sport in Diabetes

Edited by

Bill Burr and Dinesh Nagi

Pinderfields & Pontefract Hospitals NHS Trust, Wakefield, UK

JOHN WILEY & SONS, LTD

Chichester • New York • Weinheim • Brisbane • Singapore • Toronto

National 01243 779777
International (+44) 1243 779777
e-mail (for orders and customer service enquiries): cs-books@wiley.co.uk
Visit our Home Page on http://www.wiley.co.uk
or http://www.wiley.com

Other Wiley Editorial Offices

John Wiley & Sons, Inc., 605 Third Avenue,
New York, NY 10158-0012, USA

WILEY-VCH Verlag GmbH, Pappelallee 3,
D-69469 Weinheim, Germany

Jacaranda Wiley Ltd, 33 Park Road Milton,
Queensland 4064, Australia

John Wiley & Sons (Asia) Pte Ltd, 2 Clementi Loop #02-01,
Jin Xing Distripark, Singapore 129809

John Wiley & Sons (Canada) Ltd, 22 Worcester Road,
Rexdale, Ontario M9W 1L1, Canada

Library of Congress Cataloging-in-Publication Data

Exercise and sport in diabetes / edited by Bill [William A.] Burr and Dinesh [K.] Nagi.
    p.   cm.,— (Diabetes in practice)
    Includes bibliographical references and index.
    ISBN 0-471-98496-5 (cased : alk. paper)
    1. Diabetes—Exercise therapy. 2. Sports—Physiological aspects.
    3. Exercise—Physiological effect   I. Burr, William A.   II. Nagi, Dinesh K. III. Series.
    [DNLM: 1. Diabetes Mellitus. 2. Exercise–physiology. 3. Sports.
WK 810 E96 1999]
RC661.E94E94   1999
616.4′62062—DC21
DNLM/DLC
for Library of Congress   99-32280
                                                                                          CIP

British Library Cataloguing in Publication Data

A catalogue record for this book is available from the British Library

ISBN 0-471-98496-5

Typeset in 11/13pt Palatino from the authors' disks by Techset Composition Ltd, Salisbury.
Printed and bound in Great Britain by Biddles Ltd, Guildford and King's Lynn.
This book is printed on acid-free paper responsibly manufactured from sustainable forestry, in which at least two trees are planted for each one used for paper production.

Contents

Contributors

Dr Bill Burr *Consultant Physician in Diabetes/Endocrinology, Edna Coates Diabetes Centre, Pinderfields Hospital, Wakefield WF1 4DG, UK*

Dr Alan A. Connacher *Consultant Physician, Perth Royal Infirmary, Perth PH1 1NX, UK*

Dr Jean-Jacques Grimm *Division of Endocrinology and Metabolism, University Hospital, Lausanne, 2, rue du Moulin, CH-2740 Moutier, Switzerland*

Dr Veikko Koivisto *Endocrine Research and Clinical Investigation, Lilly Research Laboratories, Lilly Forschung GmbH, Wiesingerweg 25 D-20253 Hamburg, Germany*

Elizabeth Marsden *Department of Education, Canterbury Christ Church College, Canterbury CT1 1QU, Kent, UK*

Dr Dinesh Nagi *Consultant Physician in Diabetes/Endocrinology, Edna Coates Diabetes Centre, Pinderfields Hospital, Wakefield WF1 4DG, UK*

Dr Ray Newton *Consultant Physician, Ninewells Hospital, Dundee DD1 9SY, UK*

Dennis Rewt *University of Edinburgh Outdoor Activities Centre, Edinburgh, UK*

Dr Chris Thompson *Consultant Diabetologist, Department of Diabetes, Beaumont Hospital, PO Box 1297, Dublin 9, Republic of Ireland*

Professor Clyde Williams *Professor of Sports Science, Department of Physical Education, Sports Science and Recreation Management, John Hardie Building, Loughborough University, Loughborough LE11 3TU, UK*

Foreword

Anyone setting out to write a book on diabetes and exercise must come to grips with the fact that the risks and benefits are very different for the two types. The editors are to be congratulated for having got the balance right.

Let us consider the type 2 diabetes problem first. In 1997, it was calculated that it affected 124 million people in the world, and this is expected to rise to 221 million by 2010.[1] The numbers are startling but the conclusion, that this epidemic is due to a deficiency of physical exercise, is not new. In the *Medical Annual* of 1897, the Birmingham physician, Robert Saundby, wrote that, "Diabetes is undoubtedly rare among people who lead a laborious life in the open air, while it prevails chiefly with those who spend most of their time in sedentary indoor occupations", and the next year he added, "There is no doubt that diabetes must be regarded as one of the penalties of advanced civilisation". The real question is what can we do about it. Thomas McKeown[2] and others have suggested that we should stop research into the minutiae of genetics and put all our money into preventive medicine and public health, and it is certainly true that effective action will only come in the public health arena with government support. It has also been suggested that we should return to palaeolithic patterns of food and physical activity[3], and we know from O'Dea's classical experiment in returning acculturated aborigines to a traditional lifestyle, that this would work.[4] It is, however, difficult to imagine people willingly dispensing with their cars and convenience food. For the next few decades, I think the only practical solution is for the problem to be tackled on a local basis by diabetes care teams, which is why they need to read this book.

The problem in type 1 diabetes is entirely different. I agree with Dr Grimm (Chapter 2) that exercise is not a tool for improving blood glucose control, and that its benefits relate to the cardiovascular system (unproven) and to bolstering self esteem by allowing participation in a more normal lifestyle. Hopefully diabetes care teams who have read this book will help their patients avoid the experience of the tennis player, Billy Talbert.[5] He explained that when entering his first tennis tournament in 1932 at age 16:

> I had to go on and explain about the diabetes. It took some talking on my part to persuade her that I was fit to enter her husband's tournament and even then she kept eyeing me as if she expected me to drop at any moment. Her husband relieved her—and discomfited me—by promising to have a doctor at the courts.

What is really useful about this book is the wealth of practical advice, which is available in one place for the first time—previously one had to scour journal articles and back copies of *Balance* to find it. Will your patient on insulin be able to box? (No, and a jolly good thing too!) or bobsleigh down the Cresta Run? (Again, No). Most other reasonable opportunities for physical recreation are allowed and the authors explain in admirable detail how diabetic patients should prepare themselves. This is an excellent book which should be on the shelves in every diabetic clinic.

Robert Tattersall
Special Professor of Metabolic Medicine,
University of Nottingham, UK

REFERENCES

1. Amos AF, McCarty DJ, Zimmet P. The rising global burden of diabetes and its complications: estimates and projections to the year 2010. *Diabetic Medicine* 1997; **14**: S7–S85
2. McKeown T. *The origins of human disease.* Oxford: Blackwell Scientific Publications, 1988
3. Eaton SB, Shostak M, Konner M. *The Palaeolithic Prescription: a program of diet and exercise and a design for living.* New York: Harper and Row, 1988
4. O'Dea K. Marked improvement in carbohydrate and lipid metabolism in diabetic Australian Aborigines after temporary reversion to traditional lifestyle. *Diabetes* 1984; **33**: 596–603
5. Talbert WF, Sharnick J. *Playing for life.* Boston and Toronto, Little Brown and Co, 1958

Preface

Exercise, sport and physical activity pose a number of problems for professionals involved in the care of people with diabetes. On the one hand, there are increased numbers of people with type 1 diabetes. Their disease management may not be improved by playing sport and taking exercise, but it is entirely appropriate that they should be helped to take part in any sports that they may wish, in order to live life to the full. Health professionals need to be well informed to help them to do this while experiencing as little disruption as possible to daily life, and maintaining optimal levels of diabetic control to minimise the risk of complications.

These problems are entirely different from those encountered in the management of people with type 2 diabetes. We believe that a global epidemic of type 2 diabetes has begun, which will prove to be one of the biggest health challenges of the twenty-first century. The global prevalence of type 2 diabetes will have doubled in the decade 1990–2000 to an estimated 160 million, and the social and economic burdens of this will be enormous. Developing countries are being particularly affected and the costs of chronic microvascular and macrovascular complications are likely to be devastating. Various factors probably contribute to the current epidemic, and are the subject of considerable debate. Genetic, intrauterine and neonatal factors almost certainly have major effects, but the overwhelming importance of environmental factors such as age, obesity and physical inactivity cannot be denied. Obesity and physical inactivity are inextricably linked and are both potentially reversible and preventable by appropriate interventions.

There is evidence to suggest that the inexorable year-on-year rise in the prevalence of obesity in developed countries is not due to an overall increase in calorie intake but is more likely to be due to a decline in physical activity. This leads us to believe that type 2 diabetes should be regarded as a deficiency state, with the deficiency being that of physical activity.

The challenge to those of us involved in diabetes care in the twenty-first century will be to devise effective strategies to promote increased activity and physical fitness at the level of communities, as well as at the individual level. Interventions at individual level will have to be targeted at those with risk factors such as family history, ethnicity, gestational diabetes, obesity, hypertension, and impaired glucose tolerance.

We hope that this book will provide arguments to support the need for increased resources to help diabetes teams tackle the lifestyle problems of people with type 2 diabetes. We hope also that it will aid the health professional faced with the need to provide people with type 1 or 2 diabetes detailed advice to help them exercise safely and with maximum enjoyment.

Acknowledgement

We would like to acknowledge the tremendous help given by Margaret Ward from the Postgraduate Medical Centre at Pinderfields Hospital in the preparation and proof reading of this book.

1

Physiological Responses to Exercise

CLYDE WILLIAMS
Loughborough University, UK

INTRODUCTION

Exercise presents a challenge to human physiology in general and to muscle metabolism in particular. How we meet these challenges depends on the exercise intensity, its duration, our fitness and nutritional status. The aim of this chapter is to present an overview of the physiological responses to exercise which support muscle metabolism. The descriptions of carbohydrate metabolism during exercise and recovery are based on studies in non-diabetic, active individuals. The ways in which exercise affects carbohydrate metabolism in people with diabetes are discussed in Chapters 2 and 3, and in earlier reviews on this topic[1,2].

MAXIMAL EXERCISE

As we walk, cycle or run faster, there is a parallel increase in oxygen consumption ($\dot{V}O_2$) due to aerobic metabolism, which is related to exercise intensity. This linear relationship between aerobic metabolism and exercise intensity holds true for most forms of physical activity.

Exercise and Sport in Diabetes. Edited by Bill Burr and Dinesh Nagi.
© 1999 John Wiley & Sons Ltd.

Oxygen uptake continues to increase with exercise intensity until the maximum rate of oxygen consumption is reached ($\dot{V}O_2$max). Exercise can be continued at a higher intensity for a short while, without any further increase in oxygen uptake (Figure 1.1).

Maximum oxygen uptake is usually determined during exercise on a treadmill or cycle ergometer. Exercise intensity is increased step by step, either with short breaks between each stage or continuously to the point where the subject feels fatigue. There are field tests that can be used to estimate $\dot{V}O_2$max, which do not require extensive and expensive laboratory equipment. One such method is a multi-stage shuttle running test which requires only a tape recorder and a 20 m space to perform the running test[3]. It is a test which is acceptable for untrained and trained people and requires little skill to perform and evaluate.

The size of an individual's $\dot{V}O_2$max is determined by several factors, the most prominent of which are age, sex, height, weight, habitual level of physical activity, and inherited factors[4]. The genetic constitution is by far the most important influence on the maximum

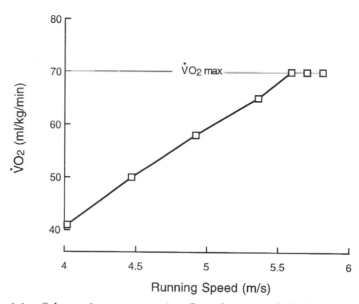

Figure 1.1. Schematic representation (based on actual data) of the relationship between the oxygen cost (ml/kg/min) of running on a level treadmill and running speed (m/s) during the assessment of an athlete's maximum oxygen uptake $\dot{V}O_2$max.

Table 1.1. The Fick Equation

Fick equation
$\dot{V}O_2$ = Heart rate × stroke volume × arteriovenous oxygen difference

Rest
$0.25\,l/min\ (\dot{V}O_2) = 5.0\,l/min\ (\dot{Q}) \times 50\,ml/l\ (A\text{-}v\ O_2)$

Maximal exercise:
Athletes $5.0\,l/min\ (\dot{V}O_2max) = 30\,l/min^{-1}\ (\dot{Q}(max)) \times 166\,ml/l^{-1}\ (A\text{-}v\ O_2)$
Active $3.0\,l/min^{-1}\ (\dot{V}O_2max) = 22\,l/min^{-1}\ (\dot{Q}(max)) \times 136\,ml/l^{-1}\ (A\text{-}v\ O_2)$

---

amount of oxygen a person can use during exercise, contributing up to 90% of an individual's $\dot{V}O_2max$[5]. However, most people, other than endurance athletes, do not get even close to their genetic limit for $\dot{V}O_2max$. The amount of physical work that people can accomplish is largely dictated by the size of their $\dot{V}O_2max$. This relationship is certainly true for runners competing in long-distance races[6,7]. Elite endurance athletes can increase their oxygen uptake from resting values of about $0.25\,l/min$ to peak values of $5.0\,l/min$ during maximum exercise lasting 2–3 minutes.

The key elements in the oxygen transport system are described by the Fick equation (see Table 1.1). Resting values for cardiac output, arteriovenous oxygen difference and oxygen uptake are similar for sedentary and well trained individuals. However, well trained athletes have maximum cardiac outputs in excess of $30\,l/min$[8], which allows them to increase their oxygen consumption by 20-fold above resting values, whereas active but not well trained individuals can achieve a 12-fold increase in their oxygen uptake values during maximum exercise.

Maximum oxygen uptake varies with age, reaching a peak in the second decade of life and decreasing thereafter[4]. The rate of decline in $\dot{V}O_2max$ is greatest in those people who take little daily exercise and least in those who maintain a good level of physical activity throughout their lives[9].

SUBMAXIMAL EXERCISE

The physiological responses to submaximal exercise are not simply proportional to, for example, walking, running, cycling or swimming speeds, but to the *relative exercise intensity*. The relative exercise intensity is defined as the oxygen cost of an activity expressed as a percentage of the individual's maximum oxygen uptake (%$\dot{V}O_2$max).

ENDURANCE TRAINING

Training improves oxygen delivery by increasing stroke volume (the amount of blood pumped with each heartbeat). This, in turn, increases maximum cardiac output without major changes in maximum heart rate, which remains unchanged or may even decrease. Training also increases the absolute amount of haemoglobin in the blood (but not the concentration). Therefore it is not unusual for athletes to have haemoglobin concentrations at the lower end of the normal range[10]. The apparent reduction in haemoglobin concentration with training is a consequence of a relatively greater increase in plasma volume than haemoglobin content[11].

Training also increases the capillary density around individual muscle fibres, and so the delivery of oxygen to muscle becomes more efficient[12]. An increase in the mitochondrial density in muscle enables greater oxygen extraction during exercise, and increases the endurance capacity of an individual during submaximal exercise, without producing changes in maximum oxygen uptake. A contributory factor to the improved exercise tolerance may be an increased capacity of trained muscle to extract oxygen from blood, which allows a decreased skeletal muscle blood flow during submaximal exercise[13,14]. This cardiovascular response to exercise, along with an increase in the aerobic metabolism of fatty acids for energy provision, and hence reduction in the formation of lactic acid, explains the improvements in exercise capacity after training.

MUSCLE FIBRE COMPOSITION

Skeletal muscles contain two main types of muscle fibres: the fast contracting, fast fatiguing fibres (Type II) and the slow contracting, slow fatiguing fibres (Type I). The rapidly contracting Type II fibres generate the energy source, adenosine triphosphate (ATP), mainly by the breakdown of their glycogen stores (glycogenolysis). In addition to the rapid formation of ATP, they also produce lactic acid, or more correctly lactate and hydrogen ions. The accumulation of hydrogen ions in Type II muscle fibres contributes to the onset of fatigue during sprinting. Training improves the aerobic capacity of these fibres, such that oxidative metabolism of glycogen makes a greater contribution to the production of ATP.

In contrast, the slow contracting, slow fatiguing Type I fibres generate ATP by the oxidative metabolism of fatty acids, glucose and glycogen. The larger oxidative capacity of these fibres is the result of their greater mitochondrial density and better oxygen utilisation than the Type II fibres. The skeletal muscles of elite marathon runners contain more Type I fibres than Type II fibres and the converse is true for top-class sprinters[15]. The marathon runner who has only a small percentage of Type II fibres may, of course, be beaten in a sprint to the finishing line by a competitor with a greater proportion of Type II fibres.

During exercise of increasing intensity, the Type I fibres are recruited first, followed by Type II fibres. This conclusion has been drawn from histochemical examination of the glycogen depletion patterns in cross-sections of active muscle fibres[16,17]. Athletes who undertake training which is mainly of low intensity and long duration will not fully recruit, and hence train, their Type II fibres. Sprinting recruits both populations of fibres because a large muscle mass is needed to generate high speeds. However, one of the limitations to maximum sprint speed is the slower speeds of Type I muscle fibres.

MUSCLE METABOLISM DURING EXERCISE

Both the respiratory and cardiovascular systems act in concert to provide working muscles with an adequate supply of oxygen for aerobic metabolism. Within the muscle cells, mitochondria produce ATP for contractile activity between the neighbouring elements, actin and myosin. In addition, the resting requirements of all cells are sustained by the continual provision of ATP, reflected by the resting metabolic rate. Oxygen is the final step in the complex process of oxidative phosphorylation that regenerates ATP from adenosine diphosphate (ADP). Some ATP is also generated by the phosphorylation of ADP from phosphocreatine (PCr). The first step in the degradation of muscle glycogen to produce ATP does not require oxygen and so is described as anaerobic glycogenolysis. Glycogenolysis provides some ATP rapidly, but only for a short time.

ANAEROBIC AND LACTATE THRESHOLDS

The accumulation of blood lactate during submaximal exercise has been interpreted as indicating that the oxygen supply to working muscles is inadequate, so there is a need for anaerobic glycogenolysis to contribute to ATP production[18]. The lactate and hydrogen ions diffuse into the venous circulation where the hydrogen ions are buffered by plasma bicarbonate. As a result of this 'bicarbonate reaction', there is an increase in carbon dioxide production which stimulates a rise in pulmonary ventilation[19,20]. This change in the rate of pulmonary ventilation has been proposed as a method of detecting the 'anaerobic threshold' or ventilatory threshold[18], which also may correlate with a rise in blood lactate[21,22].

Not everyone supports the concept of an anaerobic or ventilatory threshold. Lactate production occurs in skeletal muscle under fully aerobic conditions[23,24], and this supports the view that lactate accumulation during exercise simply reflects an increased contribution of glycogenolysis to ATP production, rather than an inadequate supply of oxygen. However, a working definition of the anaerobic or lactate threshold is as follows: during exercise of increasing intensity, a point is reached where the aerobic provision of ATP is no longer sufficient to cover the demands of working muscles and so the anaerobic production of ATP increases to complement the existing oxidative production of ATP.

Rather than attempt to detect the precise lactate thresholds of an individual, as part of a routine fitness assessment, lactate reference values are often used. For example, a blood lactate concentration of 4 mmol/l has been described as the 'onset of blood lactate accumulation' (OBLA). This particular concentration represents, for many individuals, the beginning of a steep rise in blood lactate during exercise of increasing intensity[25]. It has been proposed that the 'aerobic' and 'anaerobic' thresholds occur at blood lactate concentrations of around 2 mmol/l and 4 mmol/l respectively[26]. Even though this is an over-simplification, these lactate concentrations provide useful reference points for the routine physiological assessment of the training status of sportsmen and women[27].

An analysis of poor exercise tolerance of an individual must take into consideration whether or not the activity level is above or below the individual's anaerobic or lactate thresholds. Fatigue will occur earlier in those people who have low anaerobic thresholds than for those who have higher anaerobic thresholds[28]. The anaerobic or lactate threshold values of active people are usually expressed as a percentage of their $\dot{V}O_2$max[29], and are calculated, for instance, during submaximal running on a treadmill. Subjecting less active people, such as those recovering from illness, to heavy exercise as a means of determining their $\dot{V}O_2$max is unacceptable. Nevertheless, their functional capacity can be assessed by determining, for example, the walking speed at which their blood lactate reaches a concentration of 2 mmol/l. Monitoring this value during rehabilitation provides an objective way of following the increasing fitness of patients receiving treatment. The anaerobic or lactate threshold has proved to be a useful way of assessing the functional capacity (training status) of a person independently of their $\dot{V}O_2$max[13].

During our daily round of activities, whether they are part of work or recreation, there are only a few occasions when the contribution of glycogenolysis to energy production is greater than the contribution from aerobic metabolism of fatty acids. Running for a bus, or participation in sports such as rugby, hockey, tennis or squash, requires maximum activity for no more than a few seconds. Under these circumstances, about half the ATP is provided by the phosphorylation of ADP by PCr, and the other half is contributed by glycogenolysis[30]. Even so, the contribution of anaerobic ATP production to overall energy production during participation in these multiple-sprint sports is relatively small compared with the contribution from aerobic metabolism. This is because the brief periods of maximum exercise, essential as they are, are punctuated by longer periods of submaximal activity such as walking, running or resting.

Aerobic metabolism of fatty acids and glucose, and breakdown of liver and muscle glycogen, supports energy production during rest and during exercise. As submaximal exercise continues, there is an ever-increasing contribution of fatty acids to muscle metabolism which coincides with a decrease in the glycogen stores in liver and

Exercise and Sport in Diabetes

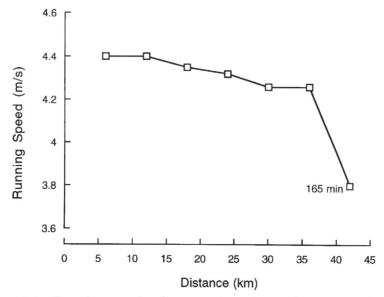

Figure 1.2. Running speeds of an experienced marathon runner during a treadmill marathon (42.2 km), during which the runner adjusted his own speed in order to achieve as fast a time as possible for this simulated race

active skeletal muscles. This shift in substrate metabolism is clearly illustrated during a treadmill marathon race (Figure 1.2).

As can be seen in Figure 1.3, carbohydrate oxidation decreases as the race continues whereas fat oxidation increases. At about 35 km, fat and carbohydrate oxidation make equal contributions to energy metabolism, and racing speed is reduced (Williams unpublished data). The reduction in running speed may be a consequence of an inability of the carbohydrate stores to continue to fuel ATP production at the rate required to maintain the initial running speed. The point in the race at which runners are forced to reduce their running speed has been described as 'hitting the wall' (see Figure 1.2).

FATIGUE AND CARBOHYDRATE METABOLISM

As the glycogen stores are gradually used up during prolonged exercise, ATP resynthesis cannot keep pace with ATP demands within each of the active muscle fibres. Even with a contribution

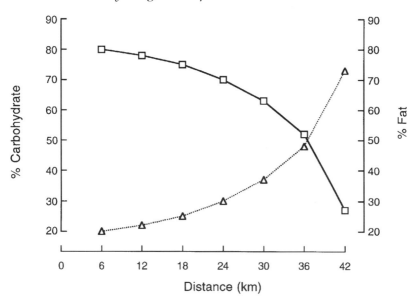

Figure 1.3. Relative contributions of carbohydrate (□) and fat (△) to energy metabolism during a treadmill marathon race (values are estimated from directly determined non-protein respiratory exchange ratios)

from intramuscular triglycerides, the high rate of ATP turnover during heavy exercise can be sustained only for as long as there is a sufficient supply of glycogen. Liver glycogen contributes to muscle metabolism via the provision of blood glucose but the delivery of this substrate is insufficient to replace the dwindling glycogen stores. When skeletal muscle glycogen concentrations reach critically low values, then exercise intensity cannot be maintained. Fatigue, under these circumstances, is clearly associated with the depletion of muscle glycogen stores. To combat this, it is not surprising that dietary manipulations have been developed to increase the body's carbohydrate stores in preparation for prolonged exercise, as well as to delay the depletion of muscle glycogen stores during prolonged exercise.

Helge *et al.* in 1998[31,32] investigated the effects of high-fat and high-carbohydrate diets on endurance capacity during cycling to exhaustion. The subjects ate a diet which provided them with either 62% of their daily energy intake from fat or 65% from carbohydrates. They continued training for 7 weeks in total, and were tested after 4 and 7 weeks. The endurance capacity of the group on a high-carbohydrate diet was significantly greater than that of the group on the high-fat diet. Even if there are some benefits to be gained from a high-fat diet before exercise, the long-term disadvantages to the health of the individual must be weighed against possible short-term gains in endurance performance.

CARBOHYDRATE NUTRITION AND EXERCISE

In developed countries, carbohydrates provide between 40 and 50% of the daily energy intake of the population, whereas in developing countries carbohydrates contribute significantly more to daily energy intake[33]. Sedentary people who become active tend to increase their daily carbohydrate intake[34]. Sportsmen and women consume more carbohydrate than the population at large[35], but even they may not eat enough to replace the carbohydrate used during daily training or competition[36–38].

Athletes undertaking heavy daily training over prolonged periods benefit from a carbohydrate intake of between 60 and 70% of their daily energy intake[36]. Most sportspeople obtain between 50 and 60% of their daily energy intake from carbohydrates and adopt nutritional strategies to achieve high carbohydrate stores before and after heavy exercise or competition.

DIETARY CARBOHYDRATE LOADING

In preparation for competition, most athletes taper their training in the week leading up to the event. Eating more carbohydrate during the 3–4 days before the competition is sufficient to increase muscle and liver glycogen stores to levels which are above normal values[39]. The recommended amount of carbohydrate is about 600 g a day (based on studies only in men). This amount of carbohydrate is clearly too great for women because it would account for almost the whole of their daily energy intake. A more helpful recommendation is one which is based on body mass, for example, 8–10 g/kg body mass per day for the 3–4 days before competition.

Dietary carbohydrate loading before cycling to exhaustion improves endurance capacity when compared with performances after a mixed diet. Early studies on carbohydrate loading reported improvements of 50% in cycling time to exhaustion[40], and the benefits of carbohydrate loading on endurance capacity during cycling have been confirmed repeatedly[41]. There have been relatively few studies on the effect of a high-carbohydrate diet on running performance, but Goforth and colleagues were amongst the first to report an improvement in endurance capacity of runners (9%) after carbohydrate loading[42]. Improvements in endurance running capacity of about 25% were also reported for male and female runners when they consumed a high-carbohydrate diet during the 3 days before a series of treadmill runs to exhaustion. One group supplemented their diet with simple carbohydrates (confectionery), and another group supplemented their diet with complex carbohydrates (pasta, potatoes and rice); the type of carbohydrate used had no influence on the subsequent improvement in endurance running capacity. Simply increasing energy intake in the form of additional protein and fat did not result in an improvement in endurance running capacity of a third group, confirming the importance of carbohydrate intake for improved performance[43].

Competitors in a 30-km cross-country race clearly benefited from dietary carbohydrate loading during the 3–4 days leading up to this endurance competition. Ten runners completed the cross-country course on two occasions separated by 3 weeks[44]. On one occasion, five of the ten runners ran the race after carbohydrate loading while the others maintained their normal mixed diets. On the second occasion the runners swapped dietary preparations and were paid to match or improve on their performance times for the first race. All the runners improved their times for the 30 km following preparation on the high-carbohydrate diet (135 min versus 143 min). This is probably the most informative study published on the influence of carbohydrate loading on running performance because not only was the study conducted as part of a real competition but also muscle biopsy samples were obtained from the runners before and after both races.

The high-carbohydrate diet for 3 days before the race significantly increased the pre-competition muscle glycogen stores. Furthermore, the carbohydrate-loaded runners completed the race in shorter times and without such a pronounced reduction in muscle glycogen as in the race preceded by the mixed diet. It is clear from this and later studies that the size of the carbohydrate stores alone will not dictate the outcome of an endurance race. Pre-race muscle glycogen stores must be sufficient to meet the demands placed on them by the endurance race; however, the benefits of carbohydrate stores in excess of this amount have not been established. Although absolute proof is lacking, the current practice is to raise carbohydrate stores as high as possible, within the constraints of time, training and dietary preparation. Other than a slight gain in body mass, there appear to be no disadvantages to dietary carbohydrate loading.

In races over shorter distances, high pre-competition muscle glycogen concentrations do not appear to improve performance. For example, there were no differences in performance times for a 20.9-km race, on an indoor 200-m track, when well trained runners consumed either a mixed diet or a high-carbohydrate diet 3–4 days before the race[39].

In contrast, starting exercise with a less than adequate glycogen store will significantly reduce exercise capacity, as has been demonstrated in laboratory studies[40,45,46]. In real competitions, such as in a soccer match, those players who began the game with low muscle glycogen concentrations ran less than the rest of the team throughout the match[47].

Most of the studies on the influences of dietary carbohydrate loading on exercise capacity have used men as subjects and some studies have failed to show the same benefits for women. It has been suggested that females use more fat for energy metabolism during submaximal exercise than males[48].

PRE-EXERCISE MEALS

Eating before competition presents a problem for many people because they feel uncomfortable when they exercise shortly after a meal. The standard advice offered is to try to eat a high-carbohydrate meal, which is easy to digest, about 3 h before exercise. However, the description of carbohydrates as either simple or complex is an inadequate way of classifying them, because not all carbohydrates produce the same metabolic response. A more informative way of classifying carbohydrates is based on the degree to which they raise blood glucose concentrations. Carbohydrates which produce a large increase in blood glucose concentration, in response to a standard amount of carbohydrate (50 g), are classified as having a high glycaemic index[49]. Table 1.2 presents a selection of foods and their glycaemic indices. The metabolic responses during exercise are influenced by the glycaemic indices of the carbohydrates in the preceding meals[50], and so the choice of carbohydrate in pre-competition meals could have an effect on performance.

Table 1.2. Glycaemic indices of common foods

Breads and grains:		Fruits:		milk, full fat	27
waffle	76	watermelon	72	milk, skimmed	32
doughnut	76	pineapple	66		
bagel	72	raisins	64	**Snacks:**	
wheat bread, white	70	banana	53	rice cakes	82
bread, wholewheat	69	grapes	52	jelly beans	80
cornmeal	68	orange	43	graham crackers	74
bran muffin	60	pear	36	corn chips	73
rice, wheat	56	apple	36	life savers	70
rice, instant	91			angel food cake	67
rice, brown	55	**Starchy vegetables:**		wheat crackers	67
rice, bulgur	48	potatoes, baked	83	popcorn	55
spaghetti, white	41	potatoes, instant	83	oatmeal cookies	55
spaghetti, wholewheat	37	potatoes, mashed	73	potato chips	54
wheat kernels	41	carrots	71	chocolate	49
barley	25	sweet potatoes	54	banana cake	47
		green peas	48	peanuts	14
Cereals:					
Rice Krispies	82	**Legumes:**		**Sugars:**	
Grape Nuts Flakes	80	baked beans	48	honey	73
Corn Flakes	77	chick peas	33	sucrose	65
Cheerios	74	butter beans	31	lactose	46
Shredded Wheat	69	lentils	29	fructose	23
Grape Nuts	67	kidney beans	27		
Life	66	soy beans	18	**Beverages:**	
Oatmeal	61			soft drinks	68
All Bran	42	**Dairy:**		orange juice	57
		ice cream	61	apple juice	41
		yoghurt, sweetened	33		

Foods listed from highest to lowest glycaemic index within category. Glycaemic index was calculated using glucose as the reference with an index of 100 (from refs 76 and 77).

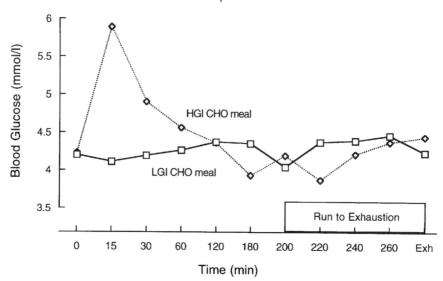

Figure 1.4. Blood glucose concentrations (mmol/l) before and after a high (HGI) and low (LGI) glycaemic carbohydrate meal and during treadmill running to exhaustion (reproduced by permission from ref. 78)

There is conflicting evidence as to whether eating high- or low-glycaemic-index foods has any effect on endurance capacity.

Figures 1.4 and 1.5 show the metabolic responses to isocaloric meals of 850 calories containing either potatoes as high-glycaemic-index or lentils as low-glycaemic-index foods, taken 3 h before treadmill exercise. Even though there were differences in the metabolic responses during the early part of exercise, there were no differences in the running times to exhaustion[78]. Nevertheless, a pre-exercise meal containing low-glycaemic-index carbohydrates may be of considerable advantage to sportsmen and women who have diabetes, because these foods lead to very little change in circulating glucose and insulin during the hours leading up to exercise.

PRE-EXERCISE DRINKS

Drinking before exercise helps to delay the onset of severe dehydration, but the type of fluid taken should be chosen with care. Water empties from the stomach quickly but crosses the walls of the small

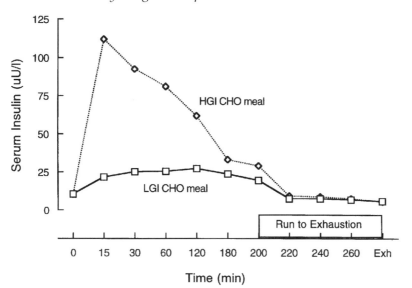

Figure 1.5. Serum insulin concentrations (μU/l) before and after a high (HGI) and low (LGI) glycaemic carbohydrate meal and during treadmill running to exhaustion (Wee *et al.*, unpublished data reproduced by permission)

intestine only slowly. Adding sodium salts to water speeds up the transport of water into the systemic circulation because of the active transport of sodium. Adding some glucose also improves the absorption of fluid, but if the glucose solution is too concentrated then gastric emptying is delayed[51]. Commercially available carbohydrate–electrolyte solutions (sports drinks) with a concentration within the range 5–8% carbohydrate appear to be most effective at supplying both fluid and fuel. The gastric emptying rate of a solution is also influenced by the volume of fluid ingested. Other things being equal, a large volume empties more quickly from the stomach than a smaller volume[52]. One strategy for rapid rehydration is to drink about 120–150 ml of fluid every 15–20 min so that the volume in the stomach does not fall to the point where emptying rate slows down.

Drinking carbohydrate–electrolyte solutions before exercise does produce, during exercise, rapid rises in blood glucose and insulin concentrations, followed by a sharp fall in blood glucose. However, as exercise continues, blood glucose concentrations normally return to pre-exercise values. It is interesting to note that, even on the occasions when blood glucose concentrations fall to hypoglycaemic values during the early part of prolonged exercise, the subjects in these studies do not report any adverse sensations[53]. In summary, the weight of the available evidence does not support the commonly held view that drinking glucose solutions before exercise leads to a reduction in exercise capacity. Nevertheless, concentrated glucose solutions (10–25%) are not recommended as a means of increasing carbohydrate stores within the hour before exercise because of the potential for causing gastrointestinal discomfort.

CARBOHYDRATE INTAKE DURING EXERCISE

Drinking carbohydrate–electrolyte solutions immediately before and throughout exercise does not produce the same fall in blood glucose as that which occurs when the same solution is ingested within the hour before exercise. One of the reasons for this different response is the failure of insulin to increase in response to the elevated blood glucose during exercise because the release of insulin from the pancreas is suppressed by the exercise-induced rise in plasma catecholamines[54]. Drinking carbohydrate–electrolyte solutions throughout prolonged exercise provides fluid and fuel, and so helps to delay the onset of severe dehydration and glycogen depletion[55–57].

The improvement in endurance capacity following the ingestion of carbohydrate–electrolyte throughout exercise has been attributed to an increased rate of carbohydrate oxidation while maintaining normal blood glucose concentrations[58]. More recent studies, using running rather than cycling, show that ingesting glucose–electrolyte solutions exerts a glycogen-sparing effect and this may be the underlying reason for the improvements in performance (for review see ref. 59)

CARBOHYDRATE INTAKE AND RECOVERY FROM EXERCISE

Rapid recovery from heavy training or competition is particularly important to sportsmen and women who have to perform every day for several days or weeks, and it is essential that they adopt a nutritional strategy which will aid rapid recovery. Central to the recovery process is the restoration of muscle and liver glycogen stores, which may have been severely depleted during exercise.

Immediately after exercise, muscle begins resynthesising the glycogen used up during exercise. The maximum rate of glycogen resynthesis occurs during the first few hours of recovery, and so ingesting carbohydrate during this period capitalises on this process. Ivy suggested that in order to maximise the glycogen resynthesis rate, the optimum post-exercise carbohydrate intake should be about 1 g/kg body mass[60]. The practical prescription is 50 g of carbohydrate immediately after exercise and the same amount every 2 h up to the next meal[61]. Depleted muscle glycogen stores can be repleted in 24 h when a carbohydrate-rich diet is eaten during the recovery period[62,63]. This recovery diet should consist of 8–10 g carbohydrate/kg body mass, and should contain high-glycaemic-index carbohydrates during at least the early part of recovery.

The key question, however, is whether or not performance capacity is restored along with muscle glycogen stores following high carbohydrate refeeding, and several studies have addressed this problem. The results suggest that as long as carbohydrate intake is increased from about 6 g/kg body mass per day to 9 g/kg, then endurance capacity is restored along with muscle glycogen stores[64].

Even when the recovery period is only a few hours, and so too short to significantly increase muscle glycogen stores, there are benefits to be gained from drinking carbohydrate–electrolyte solutions. For example, Fallowfield and colleagues reported that when runners drank a commercially available sports drink which provided the equivalent of 1 g/kg body mass of carbohydrate immediately after prolonged exercise, and again after 2 h, they were able to run for about 60 min, whereas after drinking a sweet placebo they were able to run for only 40 min[65]. Furthermore, drinking a carbohydrate–electrolyte solution is a more effective rehydrating strategy than drinking water during recovery from exercise[66].

The work of Kiens[67] and Burke[68] has shown that the type of carbohydrate eaten during recovery affects the glycogen resynthesis rate. High-glycaemic-index foods stimulate glycogen resynthesis to a greater than low-glycaemic-index foods. Adding some protein to the carbohydrate solution increases the rate of post-exercise glycogen synthesis to a greater extent than can be achieved with a carbohydrate solution alone[69]. The addition of protein increases the concentration of plasma insulin to a greater extent than when only a carbohydrate solution is consumed after exercise. An increased insulin concentration will not only increase the transport of glucose into muscle cells but will also help to restore the potassium balance across muscle membranes. However, the optimum concentrations of protein and carbohydrate for rapid glycogen resynthesis have yet to be established.

Glucose uptake by muscle is greater after exercise than before exercise. Exercise changes the characteristics of the muscle membrane so that glucose permeability is improved and muscles have an increased insulin sensitivity. The two effects appear to be additive[70]. In addition, glycogen synthase, the enzyme complex responsible for glycogen synthesis, is in its most active form immediately after exercise. There is an inverse relationship between muscle glycogen concentration and the amount of glycogen synthase in the active form[71,72], and athletes with the lowest post-exercise muscle glycogen concentrations show the greatest increase over the next 24 h[73].

More recent studies have shown that the increase in post-exercise glucose uptake is associated with an increase in the glucose transporter protein, GLUT 4, after exercise[74]. Training brings about an increase in the amount of GLUT 4 (by about 50%) with a parallel increase in the activity of hexokinase. It is probable that the rapid uptake of glucose is mainly the result of the presence of an increased amount of glucose transporter proteins[75]. These may enable an increase in the rate of glycogen resynthesis to occur, even when glycogen synthase levels have fallen to pre-exercise values.

SUMMARY

This chapter has presented a brief overview of the relevant evidence behind the nutritional strategies which are currently used by sportsmen and women in preparation for participation in, and recovery from, sport and exercise. For those people who are preparing for a prolonged period of heavy exercise, whether it is training or competition, then the recommendation is clear; they should taper their training during the week before the event and increase the carbohydrate content of their diet such that over the 48 h before the event they consume the equivalent of 8–10 g of carbohydrate/kg body weight a day. This prescription is the same for those people who have only 24 h in which to recover between training sessions or competitions. When recovery is limited to 24 h, then the high-glycaemic-index carbohydrates are recommended immediately after exercise and for most of the recovery period. However, for longer recovery periods the type of carbohydrate consumed is not as important. One of the limitations to exercise, especially in the heat, is dehydration. Drinking well formulated carbohydrate–electrolyte solutions (some sports drinks) containing no more than about 8% carbohydrate is a good strategy to decrease the rate of dehydration during exercise and provide carbohydrate as extra fuel. The recommended amounts are of the order of 120–150 ml solution every 15–20 min. This practice improves endurance running capacity, probably by contributing to the carbohydrate metabolism in working muscles. Rehydration is more rapid when carbohydrate–electrolyte solutions, rather than water alone, are consumed because thirst is quenched before rehydration is achieved when drinking water. These solutions need not contain large amounts of carbohydrate; concentrations of up to 8% appear to work well. One further point to note for those who have only a limited time in which to recover is that they need to drink the equivalent of about 50% more fluid than the volume lost during exercise.

The question about the optimum pre-exercise meal is still unanswered but there appear to be no differences in performance as a result of consuming high- or low-glycaemic-index carbohydrate foods. However, one of the advantages of a pre-exercise meal which contains predominantly low-glycaemic-index carbohydrates is that it causes only minor perturbations of plasma glucose and insulin, and so is particularly suitable for competitors who have diabetes. Furthermore, when such meals are consumed 3–4 h before exercise they provide a sense of satiety for most of the postprandial period.

In conclusion, next to being born with the appropriate genes and undertaking the right training, a high-carbohydrate diet is one of the essential elements in the formula for success in sport and exercise.

ACKNOWLEDGEMENTS

The author gratefully acknowledges the help of Judy Brewin in the preparation of this manuscript.

REFERENCES

1. Vitug A, Schneider S, Ruderman N. Exercise and Type I Diabetes Mellitus. In: Pandolf K, ed. *Exercise and Sports Sciences Reviews*, vol. 16. New York: Macmillan Publishing Company, 1988: 285–304
2. Wallberg-Henriksson H. Exercise and diabetes mellitus. In: Holloszy J, ed. *Exercise and Sport* Sciences Reviews, vol. 22. Baltimore, USA: Williams 368
3. Ramsbottom R, Brewer B, Williams C. A progressive shuttle run test to estimate maximal oxygen uptake. *Br. J. Sports Med.* 1988; **22:** 141–144
4. Astrand P-O, Rodahk K. *Textbook of Work Physiology*, 3rd edition. London: McGraw-Hill Book Company, 1986
5. Klissouras V, Pirany F, Petit J. Adaptation to maximal effort: genetics and age. *J. Appl. Physiol.* 1973; **35:** 288–293
6. Ramsbottom R, Nute MGL, Williams C. Determinants of five kilometre running performance in active men and women. *Br. J. Sports Med.* 1987; **21:** 9–13
7. Costill DL, Thomason H, Roberts E. Fractional utilization of the aerobic capacity during distance running. *Med. Sci. Sports* 1973; **5:** 248–252
8. Ekblom B, Hermansen L. Cardiac output in athletes. *J. Appl. Physiol.* 1968; **25:** 619–625
9. Knuttgen H. Physical working capacity and physical performance. *Med. Sci. Sports* 1969; **1:** 1–8
10. Brotherhood J, Brozovic B, Pugh L. Haematological status of middle and long distance runners. *Clin. Sci. Mol. Med.* 1975; **48:** 139–145
11. Eichner E. The anemias of athletes. *Phys. Sports Med.* 1986; **14:** 123–130
12. Ingjer F. Effects of endurance training on muscle fibre ATPase activity, capillary supply and mitochondrial content in man. *J. Physiol.* 1979; **294:** 419–432
13. Clausen JP. Effect of physical training on cardiovascular adjustments to exercise in man. *Physiol. Rev.* 1977; **57:** 779–815
14. Delp MD. Differential effects of training on the control of skeletal muscle perfusion. *Med. Sci. Sports Exerc.* 1998; **30:** 361–374
15. Costill DL, Daniels J, Evans W, Fink W, Krehenbuhl G, Saltin B. Skeletal muscle enzymes and fiber composition in male and female track athletes. *J. Appl. Physiol.* 1976; **40:** 149–154
16. Gollnick P, Armstrong R, Sembrowich W, Shepherd R, Saltin B. Glycogen depletion pattern in human skeletal muscle fibers after heavy exercise. *J. Appl. Physiol.* 1973; **34:** 615–618
17. Vollestad N, Vaage O, Hermansen L. Muscle glycogen depletion patterns in Type I and subgroups of Type II fibres during prolonged severe exercise in man. *Acta Physiol. Scand.* 1984; **122:** 433–441

18. Davis JA. Anaerobic threshold: review of the concept and direction for future research. *Med. Sci. Sports Exerc.* 1985; **17**: 15–18

19. Wasserman K, MacIlroy MB. Detecting the threshold of anaerobic metabolism in cardiac patients during exercise. *Am. J. Cardiol.* 1964; **14**: 844–852

20. Wasserman K, Whipp B, Koyal SN, Beaver W. Anaerobic threshold and respiratory gas exchange during exercise. *J. Appl. Physiol.* 1973; **35**: 236–243

21. Ivy JL, Withers RT, Van Handel PJ, Elger DH, Costill DL. Muscle respiratory capacity and fiber type as determinants of the lactate threshold. *J. Appl. Physiol.* 1980; **48**: 523–527

22. Yoshida T, Nagata A, Muro M, Takuechi N, Suda Y. The validity of anaerobic threshold determination by a Douglas Bag method compared with arterial blood lactate concentration. *Eur. J. Appl. Physiol.* 1981; **46**: 423–430

23. Brooks G. Anaerobic threshold: review of the concept and directions for future research. *Med. Sci. Sports Exerc.* 1985; **17**: 22–31

24. Connett RJ, Honig CR, Gayeski TEJ, Brooks GA. Defining hypoxia: a systems view of VO_2, glycolysis, energetics and intracellular PO_2. *J. Appl. Physiol.* 1990; **68**: 833–842

25. Sjodin B, Schele R, Karlsson J, Linnarsson D, Wallensten R. The physiological background of onset of blood lactate accumulation (OBLA). In: Komi P, ed. *Exercise and Sport Biology.* (International Series in Sports Sciences vol 12) Champaign: Human Kinetics, 1982: 43–56

26. Kindermann W, Simon G, Keul J. The significance of the aerobic–anaerobic transition for the determination of work load intensities during endurance training. *Eur. J. Appl. Physiol.* 1979; **42**: 25–34

27. Ramsbottom R, Williams C, Boobis L, Freeman W. Aerobic fitness and running performance of male and female recreational runners. *J. Sports Sci.* 1989; **7**: 9–20

28. Coyle EF, Coggan AR, Hopper MK, Walters TJ. Determinants of endurance in well-trained cyclists. *J. Appl. Physiol.* 1988; **64**: 2622–2630

29. Williams C, Brewer J, Patton A. The metabolic challenge of the marathon. *Br. J. Sports Med.* 1984; **18**: 245–252

30. Boobis LH. Metabolic aspects of fatigue during sprinting. In: Macleod D, Maughan R, Nimmo M, Reilly T, Williams C, eds. *Exercise, Benefits, Limitations and Adaptations.* London: E & FN Spon, 1987: 116–140

31. Helge J, Wulff B, Kiens B. Impact of a fat-rich diet on endurance in man: role of dietary period. *Med. Sci. Sports Exerc.* 1998; **30**: 456–461

32. Helge J, Richter E, Kiens B. Interaction of training and diet on metabolism and endurance during exercise in man. *J. Physiol.* 1996; **492**: 293–306

33. Stephen AM, Sieber GM, Gerster YA, Morgan RD. Intake of carbohydrate and its components-international comparison: trends over time, and effects of changing to a low fat diet. *Am. J. Clin. Nutr.* 1995; **62**: 851S–867S

34. Janssen G, Graef C, Saris W. Food intake and body composition in novice athletes during a training period to run a marathon. *Int. J. Sports Med.* 1989; **10** (supplement 1): S17–S21

35. Williams C. Carbohydrate needs of elite athletes. In: Simopoulos A, Pavlou K, ed. *Nutrition and Fitness of Athletes*. (Simopoulos AP, ed. World Review of Nutrition and Dietetics; vol 71) New York: Karger, 1993: 34–60

36. Devlin J, Williams C. Foods, nutrition and sports performance; a final consensus statement. *J. Sports Sci.* 1991; **9** (Suppl. 9): iii

37. Ekblom B, Williams C. Foods, nutrition and soccer performance: final consensus statement. *J. Sports Sci.* 1994; **12** (special issue): S3

38. Maughan R, Horton E. Current issues in nutrition in athletics: final consensus statement. *J. Sports Sci.* 1995; **13** (special issue): Si

39. Sherman W, Costill D, Fink W, Miller J. Effect of exercise–diet manipulation on muscle glycogen and its subsequent utilization during performance. *Int. J. Sports Med.* 1981; **2**: 114–118

40. Bergstrom J, Hermansen L, Hultman E, Saltin B. Diet, muscle glycogen and physical performance. *Acta Physiol. Scand.* 1967; **71**: 140–150

41. Conlee R. Muscle glycogen and exercise endurance: a twenty year prospective. In: Pandolf K, ed. *Exercise and Sports Science Reviews*, vol 15. London: Collier Macmillan, 1987: 1–28.

42. Goforth HW, Hodgdon JA, Hilderbrand RL. A double blind study of the effects of carbohydrate loading upon endurance performance. *Med. Sci. Sports Exerc.* 1980; **12**: 108A

43. Brewer J, Williams C, Patton A. The influence of high carbohydrate diets on endurance running performance. *Eur. J. Appl. Physiol.* 1988; **57**: 698–706

44. Karlsson J, Saltin B. Diet, muscle glycogen and endurance performance. *J. Appl. Physiol.* 1971; **31**: 203–206

45. Maughan RJ, Williams C, Campbell DM, Hepburn D. Fat and carbohydrate metabolism during low intensity exercise: effects of the availability of muscle glycogen. *Eur. J. Appl. Physiol.* 1978; **39**: 7–16

46. Maughan RJ, Poole DC. The effects of a glycogen-loading regimen on the capacity to perform anaerobic exercise. *Eur. J. Appl. Physiol.* 1981; **46**: 211–219

47. Saltin B. Metabolic fundamentals of exercise. *Med. Sci. Sports Exerc.* 1973; **15**: 366–369

48. Tarnoposky LJ, MacDougall JD, Atkinson SA, Tarnopolsky MA, Sutton

JR. Gender differences in substrate for endurance exercise. *J. Appl. Physiol.* 1990; **68:** 302–307

49. Jenkins DJA, Thomas DM, Wolever MS *et al.* Glycemic index of foods: a physiological basis for carbohydrate exchange. *Am. J. Clin. Nutr.* 1981; **34:** 362–366

50. Horowitz JF, Coyle EF. Metabolic responses to pre-exercise meals containing various carbohydrates and fat. *Am. J. Clin. Nutr.* 1993; **58:** 235–241

51. Vist G, Maughan R. Gastric emptying of ingested solutions in man: effect of beverage glucose concentration. *Med. Sci. Sports Exerc.* 1994; **26:** 1269–1273

52. Noakes TD, Rehrer NJ, Maughan RJ. The importance of volume in regulating gastric emptying. *Med. Sci. Sports Exerc.* 1991; **23:** 307–313

53. Chryssanthopoulos C, Hennessy L, Williams C. The influence of pre-exercise glucose ingestion on endurance running capacity. *Br. J. Sports Med.* 1994; **28:** 105–109

54. Porte D, Williamson R. Inhibition of insulin release by norepinephrine in man. *Science* 1966; **152:** 1248–1250

55. Murray R. Fluid needs in hot and cold environments. *Int. J. Sports Nutr.* 1995; **5:** S62–S73

56. Tzintzas O, Williams C, Boobis L, Greenhaff P. Carbohydrate ingestion and glycogen utilization in different muscle fibre types in man. *J. Physiol.* 1995; **489:** 243–250

57. Tsintzas O, Williams C, Singh R, Wilson W, Burrin J. Influence of carbohydrate–electrolyte drinks on marathon running performance. *Eur. J. Appl. Physiol.* 1995; **70:** 161–168

58. Coyle EF, Coggan AR, Hemmert MK, Ivy JL. Muscle glycogen utilization during prolonged strenuous exercise when fed carbohydrate. *J. Appl. Physiol.* 1986; **61:** 165–172

59. Tsintzas K, Williams C. Human muscle glycogen metabolism during exercise: effect of carbohydrate supplementation. *Sports Med.* 1998; **25:** 7–23

60. Ivy JL. Muscle glycogen synthesis before and after exercise. *Sports Med.* 1991; **11:** 6–19

61. Coyle E. Timing and method of increased carbohydrate intake to cope with heavy training, competition and recovery. *J. Sports Sci.* 1991; **9** (Suppl.): 29–52

62. Bergstrom J, Hultman E. Muscle glycogen synthesis after exercise: an enhancing factor localized to the muscle cell in man. *Nature* 1966; **20:** 309–310

63. Keizer H, Kuipers H, van Kranenburg G. Influence of liquid and solid meals on muscle glycogen resynthesis, plasma fuel hormone response, and maximal physical working capacity. *Int. J. Sports Med.* 1987; **8:** 99–104

64. Fallowfield J, Williams C. Carbohydrate intake and recovery from prolonged exercise. *Int. J. Sport Nutr.* 1993; **3**: 150–164

65. Fallowfield J, Williams C, Singh R. The influence of ingesting a carbohydrate–electrolyte solution during 4 hours recovery from prolonged running on endurance capacity. *Int. J. Sport Nutr.* 1995; **5**: 285–299

66. Gonzalez-Alonso J, Heaps CL, Coyle EF. Rehydration after exercise with common beverages and water. *Int. J. Sports Med.* 1992; **13**: 399–406

67. Kiens B. Translating nutrition into diet: diet for training and competition. In: Macleod DAD, Maughan RJ, Williams C, Madeley CR, Sharp JCM, Nutton RW, eds. *Intermittent High Intensity Exercise: Preparation, Stresses and Damage Limitation.* London: E & FN Spon, 1993: 175–182

68. Burke L, Collier G, Hargreaves M. Muscle glycogen storage after prolonged exercise: effect of the glycaemic index of carbohydrate feedings. *J. Appl. Physiol.* 1993; **75**: 1019–1023

69. Zawadzki K, Yaspelkis III B, Ivy J. Carbohydrate–protein complex increases the rate of muscle glycogen storage after exercise. *J. Appl. Physiol.* 1992; **72**: 1854–1859

70. Wallberg-Henriksson H, Constable SH, Young DA, Holloszy JO. Glucose transport into rat skeletal muscle: interaction between exercise and insulin. *J. Appl. Physiol.* 1988; **65**: 909–913

71. Adolfsson S, Ahren K. Control mechanisms for the synthesis of glycogen in striated muscle. In: Pernow B, Saltin B, eds. *Muscle Metabolism During Exercise.* New York: Plenum Press, 1971: 257–272

72. Piehl K, Adolfsson S, Nazar K. Glycogen storage and glycogen synthetase activity in trained and untrained muscle of man. *Acta Physiol. Scand.* 1974; **90**: 779–788

73. Jacobs I, Westlin N, Karlsson J, Rasmusson M, Houghton B. Muscle glycogen and diet in elite soccer players. *Eur. J. Appl. Physiol.* 1982; **48**: 297–302

74. McCoy M, Proietto J, Hargreaves M. Skeletal muscle Glut 4 and post-exercise muscle glycogen storage in humans. *J. Appl. Physiol.* 1996; **80**: 411–415

75. Nakatani A, Han D-H, Hansen P *et al.* Effect of endurance exercise training on muscle glycogen supercompensation in rats. *J. Appl. Physiol.* 1997; **82**: 711–715

76. Rankin WJ. Glycemic index and exercise metabolism. *Sports Sci. Exch.* 1997; **10**: 1–6

77. Foster-Powell K, Brand-Miller J. International tables of glycemic index. *Am. J. Clin. Nutr.* 1995; **62**: 871S–890S

78. Wee SL, Williams C, Gray S, Horabin J. Influence of high and low glycemic index meals on endurance running capacity. *Med. Sci. Sports Exerc.* 1999; **31**: 393–399

2

Exercise in Type 1 Diabetes

JEAN-JACQUES GRIMM
University Hospital Lausanne, Switzerland

INTRODUCTION

Regular exercise in people with type 1 diabetes does not necessarily lead to improved control. Indeed, the metabolic disturbances associated with sustained exercise may lead to worsening control unless great care is taken to adjust insulin and carbohydrate intake. Type 1 diabetes frequently affects children, adolescents and young adults in whom health improvement does not feature highly among the reasons for taking exercise. The desire to play, or to become a member of a team, is often more important, and is driven by social reasons and the need not to appear 'different' from the peer group. The aim of the medical team is to allow the diabetic child or adult to participate in the sport of his or her choice and to avoid any form of discrimination during school sports or when playing in a team.

This chapter deals with the way a person with type 1 diabetes could manage their condition independently and safely during various kinds of sports and exercises.

Recent literature[1,2] acknowledges that 'all levels of exercise, including leisure activities, recreational sports, and competitive professional activities, can be performed by people with type 1 diabetes'. It must be stressed, however, that high-intensity endurance exercise (e.g.

Exercise and Sport in Diabetes. Edited by Bill Burr and Dinesh Nagi.
© 1999 John Wiley & Sons Ltd.

marathon, triathlon, kayaking) is not required to achieve maximal health benefit from exercise. Regular, moderate-intensity exercise[1,3] has the best risk/benefit ratio.

The advantages of exercise in type 1 diabetes relate more to its protective cardiovascular effects than to improved glycaemic control. Exercise is not a tool for improving blood glucose control in type 1 diabetes, but the diabetes education team needs to be knowledgeable about all treatment adjustments required to enable their patients to exercise safely and with maximum health benefit.

EXERCISE PHYSIOLOGY

As well as an increase in oxygen availability, exercise requires rapid mobilisation and redistribution of metabolic fuels to ensure an adequate energy supply for the working muscles (see Chapter 1). This necessitates a cascade of neural, cardiovascular and hormonal adjustments.

FUELS METABOLISED BY SKELETAL MUSCLE

Skeletal muscle metabolises mainly glucose, free fatty acids (FFA) and triglycerides. Ketones do not participate in the oxidative metabolism of active muscles in healthy humans[4]. Amino acids derived from catabolism within the muscle can be used as an energy source by muscles during very long and very intense effort. Nevertheless, amino acids never contribute more than 10% to the total energy expenditure[5].

SOURCES AND PROPORTIONS OF FUELS USED DURING EXERCISE

During the first 20–30 min of effort, muscle glycogen is the main source of energy[6]. Later, blood-borne glucose derived from hepatic glycogenolysis, gluconeogenesis and intestinal absorption is metabolised, followed by muscle triglycerides and circulating FFA derived from adipose tissue (Figure 2.1).

At rest almost no blood glucose enters the muscle cell. During the first 10 min of exercise, blood glucose represents 10–15% of oxidative metabolism, and after 90 min it can increase to 40% of the total fuel

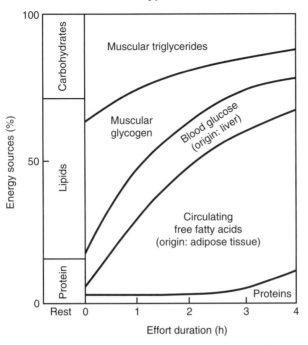

Figure 2.1. Regulation of energy sources during mild exercise of long duration. Experimental situation without glucose ingestion[7]

utilisation[8]. After 4 h of exercise, blood glucose provides approximately one-third and FFA two-thirds of the oxidative fuels[9]. After 8 h of moderate exercise, FFAs are responsible for 80–85% of the oxidative fuel, the rest being derived from glucose with a small contribution from branched-chain amino acids[10].

REGULATION OF FUEL DELIVERY DURING EXERCISE

During exercise of moderate intensity, insulin and glucagon are the main regulators of hepatic glucose production. A low level of plasma insulin is required to allow hepatic glycogenolysis, and an increase in glucagon concentration is necessary for both glycogenolysis and gluconeogenesis[11]. The glucagon/insulin ratio correlates better with hepatic glucose production than insulin or glucagon levels alone[12]. It seems that a decrease in insulin level enhances hepatic sensitivity to the action of glucagon. Without the presence of glucagon, however, the decrease in insulin concentration alone does not stimulate hepatic glycogenolysis[13].

Adrenaline stimulates hepatic glucose production during intense effort of long duration by facilitating mobilisation of the precursors of gluconeogenesis. Catecholamines are also responsible for extra glucose production during very intense exercise of short duration[14,15].

Lipolysis is stimulated by increased catecholamine levels, which also suppress insulin secretion. Increased α-adrenergic stimulation from noradrenaline released from sympathetic nerves seems to be the most prominent stimulus to lipolysis[16], together with increased sensitivity of the adipocytes to catecholamines[17].

CONSEQUENCES OF DIABETES ON THE METABOLIC RESPONSE TO EXERCISE

The problems relating to blood glucose control in physically active insulin-treated people can be explained by imbalances between the plasma insulin level and the available plasma glucose. Very often the plasma insulin, derived from injected insulin, is too high during

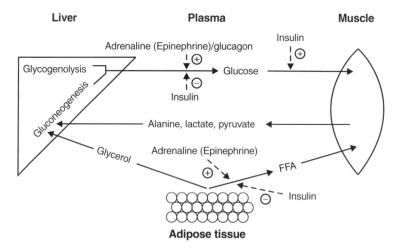

Figure 2.2. Main energy fluxes during exercise, and their regulation in blood glucose homeostasis. In the non-diabetic exercising subject, the plasma insulin level decreases whereas the adrenaline and glucagon levels increase. Adapted from ref. 18 by permission of Lilly Research Laboratories

exercise compared with the insulin level of a non-diabetic person in the same situation. At the same time, the carbohydrate supply is often too low, because hepatic glycogenolysis is blocked by high insulin levels (Figure 2.2).

INSULIN ABSORPTION

The importance of changing the injection site when doing sports or being physically active is an old and ongoing debate. Various factors speed the rate of insulin absorption, including increased blood flow to the injection site due to exercise or increased ambient temperature[19,20] and local massage[21]. There is considerable intra-individual variation in insulin absorption rate (up to 15% difference for the same site from day to day[22]), and it has been shown that insulin absorption from sites in the abdomen is significantly more rapid than from sites in the thigh. In the 1970s experimental data[23] showed that muscular activity speeds insulin absorption from an exercising limb. This was considered at least part of the explanation for the increased insulin action during exercise. Many considered that injecting the insulin into a non-exercising area would help to prevent hypoglycaemic attacks during and after exercise, but Kemmer *et al.*[24] showed that this strategy did not prevent effort-related hypoglycaemia. Because of the difference between different injection sites, we would not advocate using a different site on a one-off basis specifically for athletic activity—this would simply add another variable. Because absorption rates vary from site to site, it is sensible to restrict short-acting insulin injections to one site. If the abdomen is used routinely, this obviates the worries about varying insulin absorption rates from an exercising limb.

RISK OF INVOLUNTARY INTRAMUSCULAR INJECTION

Intramuscular injection of insulin is a cause of hypoglycaemia[25] independent of exercise. It is clear that this risk is increased if the injection is followed by exercise. The physically active diabetic person must be informed of the need to avoid intramuscular injections and to take particular care with injection technique.

Short needles (8.0 mm) have been marketed with the claim that they avoid the risk of intramuscular injection and obviate the need for pinching the skin. However, it seems that even with 8.0 mm needles some insulin injections can be intramuscular when injected without a skin fold in lean persons. Furthermore, short needles expose the patient to the risk of intradermal injections or insulin leaks when the technique is not perfect. Consequently, we suggest routinely using a skin fold when injecting insulin, whatever the length of the needle used (8.0, 10.0 or 12.7 mm).

Recommendations for exercise and insulin injections

1. Inject the insulin into the usual location.
2. Take special care with the injection to make sure it is not intramuscular.
2. Learn to adapt (decrease) the insulin dose, depending on the type, duration and timing of exercise.
4. Use frequent blood glucose measurements, especially during unfamiliar activities.

HYPOGLYCAEMIA

The risk of hypoglycaemia during exercise in the insulin-dependent diabetic person was expertly described, a few years after the discovery of insulin, by the British physician R.D. Lawrence[26]. In contrast to the non-diabetic subject, where the insulin level falls shortly after exercise commences, the insulin level in the person with diabetes is governed mainly by the amount and timing of the last injection. It follows that he or she must anticipate strenuous activities and make appropriate reductions in the insulin dose. If this is not done, the only option is to take extra carbohydrate to try to compensate for an excess of circulating insulin.

Fear of hypoglycaemic coma has often been a cause of discrimination against children with diabetes, leading to their exclusion from gymnastics or from summer camps. Some children with diabetes decide spontaneously not to participate in group or team activities, for fear of upsetting their team-mates because of the need for regular blood glucose checks and the necessity to eat snacks at precise times, or because a hypoglycaemic episode might upset the team performance.

Hypoglycaemia may happen during exercise, but also 12–14 h or even longer after the end of the effort[27,28]. Late-onset hypoglycaemia is explained both by the body's need to replenish glycogen stores and by a sustained increase of tissue sensitivity to insulin. When the exercise sessions continue for several days, insulin needs usually decrease progressively from day to day.

Repeated episodes of hypoglycaemia lead to an unfortunate vicious circle whereby there is decreased hypoglycaemic awareness, leading to the risk of more hypoglycaemia[29]. Furthermore, physical activity makes recognition of hypoglycaemia difficult because sweating and tachycardia due to physical effort can mask similar signs warning of impending hypoglycaemia.

When hypoglycaemia happens during exercise despite all efforts to avoid it, it is often extremely difficult to treat. Very often the activity has to be temporarily suspended, and the amount of carbohydrate required to correct the blood glucose may be unusually high—often 30–40 g or more. Exercise-onset hypoglycaemia tends to be recurrent and more carbohydrate may be needed within half an hour (preferably after a repeat blood glucose test).

HYPERGLYCAEMIA

Exercise can cause a rise in blood glucose in two situations: (1) when an individual is insulin deficient and metabolically unstable; (2) with extremely intense exercise in well controlled individuals.

PRE-EXERCISE HIGH BLOOD GLUCOSE AND KETONES

This situation is the consequence of a severe deficit in circulating insulin leading to an increase in hepatic glucose production, a decrease in glucose disposal by muscle, and the production of ketones. Furthermore, exercise stimulates the secretion of counter-regulatory hormones (glucagon, catecholamines, growth hormone, and cortisol), all of which contribute to hyperglycaemia and metabolic deterioration[30].

Hyperglycaemia (>14.0 mmol/l glucose) with ketonuria is an absolute contraindication to exercise. The metabolic imbalance must be corrected by short-acting insulin injections and the activity must not be resumed until the blood glucose level starts to decrease.

VERY INTENSE SHORT EXERCISE WITH NORMAL BLOOD GLUCOSE

Very intense (>80% of maximal oxygen uptake ($\dot{V}O_2$max) and short-duration exercise, such as weight-lifting, can increase glycaemia. The main explanation is a great increase in catecholamine production[15]. In the original work of Mitchell *et al.*[14], the duration of the effort was 10 min and the intensity 80% of the $\dot{V}O_2$max. Two groups of diabetics were observed, a metabolically well controlled group (mean blood glucose: 4.8 mmol/l), and a less well controlled group (mean blood glucose: 8.3 mmol/l). Two hours after exercise, the increase in blood glucose was 2.9 mmol/l in the well controlled group and 4.2 mmol/l in the less controlled group.

When short bouts of intense exercise are repeated many times during a limited time span (1–2 h) as, for example, during an ice hockey game, energy consumption is considerable, and will finally lead to a decrease in blood glucose, with a risk of hypoglycaemia.

STRATEGIES FOR TREATMENT ADJUSTMENTS

Two important principles must be taken into account in making treatment adjustments during and after exercise in people with type 1 diabetes:

1. Exercise is always associated with extra energy consumption.
2. Exercise stimulates glucose uptake into muscle cells (increases insulin sensitivity). The same amount of insulin allows more glucose to be metabolised during effort than at rest (Figure 2.3).

Most people with type 1 diabetes who are planning to exercise have heard about insulin dose adjustments before exercise and are aware of the increased risk of hypoglycaemia. However, experience shows that very often they underestimate the reduction in insulin dose required. On top of this, the need to compensate for increased energy expen-

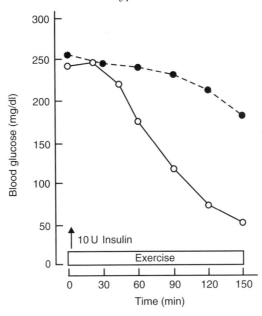

Figure 2.3. Effect of subcutaneously injected insulin at rest (●) and with muscular exercise (○)[26]

diture with extra carbohydrate is often neglected, forgotten or underestimated; this is the main cause of preventable hypoglycaemia[31].

These errors become critical when, due to an excess of circulating insulin, hepatic glycogen stores cannot be mobilised and gluconeogenesis cannot occur (see Figure 2.2).

Correct preparation for exercise needs a detailed assessment of all the characteristics of the effort: duration, intensity, time from last meal, time of day and insulin activity (blood insulin levels) during the exercise session. Frequent blood glucose measurement is of value during the first few attempts at any new activity.

- Leaving a short interval of up to 2 h between the last meal/insulin injection and exercise can give some protection against hypoglycaemia, especially when using classical insulins. This is no longer true with the very short-acting insulin analogue 'Lispro' (Humalog®), which results in higher insulin levels within 2 h of injection[32] (see Chapter 6).

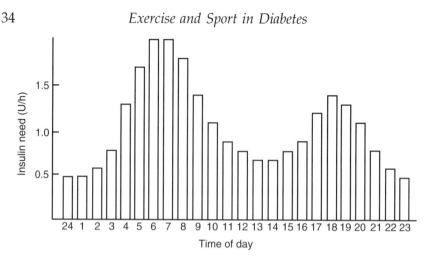

Figure 2.4. Variations of the hourly insulin needs over 24 h, independently of meals, in 198 subjects with type 1 diabetes treated by continuous subcutaneous insulin infusion pump therapy[33]

- Time of day is important, not only because insulin levels fluctuate through the day but also because the needs of the body for insulin are low at certain times of the day (Figure 2.4).
- Estimation of the times when insulin levels are high for every type of insulin injection is one of the important homework tasks for the would-be exerciser[34]. Table 2.1 shows 'intense' insulin activity periods for different insulin preparations and dosages. Exercising during these periods needs special attention because of the increased risk of hypoglycaemia. When exercise takes place during maximum activity of the background insulin, the dose of short-acting insulin may need more drastic reduction, with additional carbohydrate supplements, compared with exercise when background insulin is low.

EVALUATION OF THE INTENSITY AND DURATION OF THE EFFORT

INTENSITY

Effort intensity is well correlated with heart rate (HR) in the absence of heart rhythm abnormalities or autonomic neuropathy. One way of

Table 2.1. Periods of 'intense' insulin activity of different insulin preparations and dosages. The 'period of intense insulin activity' is defined as the time between the moment when insulin activity reaches two-thirds and the moment when it falls below two-thirds of the peak[34]

Type of insulin	Units	T 50% (hours)	Period of intense insulin (h) activity, subcutaneous injection			Period of intense insulin activity (h) after subcutaneous injection
			Start	End	Variation (end)	
Short-acting insulin analogue (Humalog® Novorapid®)	10	1.3	0.5	2.6	2.3–3.3	
Short-acting insulin (Actrapid®)	6	2.3	1	4.6	3.5–5.8	
	12	2.7	1	5.4	4.1–6.8	
	20	3.0	1	6.0	4.5–7.5	
Basal insulins: NPH	6	7.5	2.5	9.0	6.7–11.3	
	12	8.5	2.5	10.2	7.7–12.8	
	24	10.6	2.5	12.8	9.5–16.0	
	36	13.0	2.5	15.6	11.7–19.5	
Zinc insulins: Monotard HM®	6	7.3	3.0	8.8	6.6–11.0	
	12	8.9	3.0	10.7	8.8–13.4	
	24	10.9	3.0	13.1	9.8–16.4	
	36	14.8	3.0	17.8	13.3–22.3	
Ultratard HM®	6	13.0	4–6	15.6	11.7–19.5	
	24	15.1	4–6	18.1	13.6–22.6	
Semi lente®	40	8.0	2.5	12.0	9.0–15.0	

↑ s.c. injection

defining the intensity of exercise is to state the actual HR as a percentage of the maximal HR. The maximal HR can be calculated or measured during a bicycle or treadmill stress test. Calculated (theoretical) maximal HR for all women or untrained men is 220 minus age. For trained men, it is 205 minus $0.5 \times$ age[35].

Example 1: calculation of maximal HR

- Untrained 50-year-old man. Maximal HR: 220–50 = 170 beats/min.
- Trained 40-year-old man. Maximal HR: 205–20 = 185 beats/min.

Exercise intensity is defined according to the following formula:

- Low-intensity exercise:<60% of maximal HR.
- Moderate-intensity exercise: 60–75% of maximal HR.
- High-intensity exercise: >75% of maximal HR.

Example 2 estimation of exercise intensity

40-year-old woman, HR during exercise: 80 beats/min. Maximal HR: 220–40 = 180 beats/min. HR/maximal HR = 80/180 = 45%. This exercise is of low intensity.

DURATION

Short <20 min; medium 20–60 min; long >60 min.

CHARACTERISATION OF THE EFFORT

Table 2.2 shows nine combinations of different durations and intensities of exercise. Every exercise session can be characterised with this chart.

NUTRITIONAL TREATMENT ADAPTATIONS

Without energy, there can be no exercise! The energy comes from stores located in the body or from ingested food or beverages. *The*

Table 2.2. Extra carbohydrate amounts and insulin dose reductions for different sessions. The values in bold show situations where an insulin dosage reduction is required

	Duration (min)		
Intensity (% of max HR)	Short (<20)	Medium (20–60)	Long (>60)
Low (<60)	0–10 g	10–20 g	**10–20 g/h**
Moderate (60–75)	10–20 g	**20–60 g**	**20–100 g/h**
High (>75)	0–30 g	**30–100 g**	**30–100 g/h**

diabetic person relies even more than non-diabetic subjects on an adequate energy intake before, during and after exercise.

Although glucose represents only a part of the fuel metabolised during exercise, for simplification during patient education it is suggested that the energy expended must be replaced in the form of glucose, or carbohydrate equivalent, during and after exertion. People with diabetes whose insulin dosage has been adequately reduced need at least as much extra glucose during an effort as non-diabetics[36].

Carbohydrate supplementation alone will prevent most hypoglycaemic episodes[31]. Precise counselling in carbohydrate supplementation is extremely difficult, but Table 2.2 provides a guide for the approximate amounts of additional carbohydrate required for exercises of different duration and intensity. The amounts of carbohydrate have been validated in adults doing different activities (callisthenics, walking, mountain biking; personal data).

The proposed extra carbohydrate intakes are rough estimates, with relatively wide ranges. It is possible to increase the precision (make the range narrower) by comparing with the amounts listed in Table 2.3, which gives estimates of carbohydrate requirements for particular sports and activities and for three different body weights[37].

Although these tables give some indication of the energy expenditure associated with different activities and provide a starting point from which to make adjustments, at the end of the day there is no substitute for experience and for trial and (hopefully not too much) error. An important point is that the insulin plasma level at the start of exercise is never known. It can, however, be roughly estimated by observation of the slope between two blood glucose measurements at

Table 2.3.   Grams of carbohydrate used each hour in common activities[37]

Activity	Grams of CHO used per hour by weight			Approximate percentage of total calories from CHO
	100 lb (45 kg)	150 lb (68 kg)	200 lb (90 kg)	
Baseball	25	38	50	40
Basketball:				
moderate	35	53	70	50
vigorous	59	89	118	60
Bicycling:				
6 mph	20	27	34	40
10 mph	35	48	61	50
14 mph	60	83	105	60
18 mph	95	130	165	65
20 mph	122	168	214	70
Dancing:				
moderate	17	25	33	40
vigorous	28	43	57	50
Digging	45	65	83	50
Eating	6	8	10	30
Golfing (pullcart)	23	35	46	40
Handball	59	88	117	60
Jump rope 80/min	73	109	145	65
Mopping	12	18	24	30
Mountain climbing	60	90	120	60
Outside painting	21	31	42	40
Raking leaves	19	28	38	30
Running:				
5 mph	45	68	90	50
8 mph	96	145	190	65
10 mph	126	189	252	70
Shovelling	31	45	57	50
Skating:				
moderate	25	34	43	40
vigorous	67	92	117	60
Skiing:				
cross-country 5 mph	76	105	133	60
downhill	52	72	92	50
water	42	58	74	50
Soccer	45	67	89	50

Table 2.3. (*continued*)

Activity	Grams of CHO used per hour by weight			Approximate percentage of total calories from CHO
	100 lb (45 kg)	150 lb (68 kg)	200 lb (90 kg)	
Swimming:				
slow crawl	41	56	71	50
fast crawl	69	95	121	60
Tennis:				
moderate	28	41	55	40
vigorous	59	88	117	60
Volleyball:				
moderate	23	34	45	40
vigorous	59	88	117	60
Walking:				
3 mph	15	22	29	30
4.5 mph	30	45	59	45

15 and 30 min before exercise. A pronounced fall would indicate that additional carbohydrate is likely to be needed.

For endurance activities (several hours), the hourly need for extra carbohydrate will often reduce for two reasons:

1. A shift towards FFA consumption rather than glucose by the active muscle.
2. A drifting away from the period of maximal insulin action (in most cases) and decreased risk of insulin excess.

The relative amount of carbohydrate or FFA oxidised during an endurance effort will depend on the patient's fitness level. Trained athletes oxidise FFA earlier and in greater amounts than untrained athletes and will spare carbohydrates in this way.

INSULIN DOSE ADJUSTMENT

Even the most sophisticated insulin treatment scheme (subcutaneous insulin infusion pump or multiple insulin injections) cannot mimic the subtle insulin adjustments of a healthy pancreas. The most common failing of insulin therapy, compared with natural secretion, is a lack of insulin in the minutes following the start of a meal and an excess of insulin 3–4 h after the meal. These faults can partly be avoided with pump treatment or with subcutaneous injections of the new very-short-acting insulin analogue Lispro, combined with a split (divided into two or three injections during the day) basal insulin administration (see Chapter 6).

As insulin regimens and formulations differ widely from patient to patient, the strategies must be personalised. For low-intensity exercise lasting up to 1 h, and for any higher intensity exercise lasting less than 20 min, it is usually not necessary to change the insulin dose (Table 2.4). If the starting blood glucose is low or falling, it is wise to eat a snack before starting. Table 2.4 considers the insulins which are active during *and* after exercise.

Example 1: 45 minutes jogging from 2.00 to 3.00 p.m.

If taking a basal/bolus regimen, the pre-lunch soluble insulin would need to be reduced by 10–50%. If using a twice-daily regimen of

Table 2.4. Decrease in insulin dosage for efforts of different intensities and durations

Intensity	Duration (min)		
(% of max HR)	<20	20–60	>60
Low (<60): e.g. walking, slow swimming	—	—	Prandial insulin: 5–10%/h exercise Basal insulin: 5–10%/h exercise
Moderate (60–70): e.g. hiking, cycling, jogging	—	Prandial insulin: 10–50% Basal insulin: 10–20%	Prandial insulin: 5–10%/h exercise Basal insulin: 5–10%/h exercise
High (>75): e.g. mountain biking, running, competition cycling or swimming	—	Prandial insulin: 10–50% Basal insulin: 10–20%	Prandial insulin: 5–20%/h exercise Basal insulin: 5–20%/h exercise

soluble and intermediate insulin, the morning dose should not be reduced because this would cause pre-lunch hyperglycaemia. In this case the only recourse would be to take extra carbohydrate.

Example 2: 45 minutes cycling after dinner, from 7.00 to 8.00 p.m

Decrease the short-acting insulin of the dinner injection (10–50%) and basal night injection (10–20%) for those on basal/bolus and of the dinner soluble and intermediate insulins if on twice-daily injections.

Example 3: 2 hours slow swimming from 5.00 to 7.00 p.m; dinner at 7.45 p.m

Decrease the short-acting insulin of the dinner injection (5–10% × 2 = 10–20%) and basal insulin of the dinner or night injection (5–10% × 2 = 10–20%).

Example 4: Hiking or skiing from 10.00 a.m. to 1.00 p.m. and from 2.00 p.m. to 4.00 p.m. (total: 5 h)

Decrease the short-acting insulins of the lunch and dinner injections (25–50%) and basal insulins of the morning and evening injections (25–50%).

In all four examples, the insulin dosage adaptations must be combined with extra carbohydrate intake.

CONCLUSIONS

We live in a society battling against cardiovascular diseases, which are, in large part, the consequence of our lifestyles. Along with decreased usage of tobacco and more healthy eating habits, regular physical exercise is of major importance for the improvement and maintenance of health[38]. In addition, exercise is a source of pleasure and social contact for many people. It is therefore only natural that strategies have been developed which permit, and even encourage, those who have type 1 diabetes to devote themselves to the physical activity of their choice.

Before undertaking any exercise programme we would advise a general medical check-up, which should concentrate on the potential complications of diabetes, especially cardiovascular disease. This is even more important in those who have previously lived a sedentary lifestyle.

To be physically active, safe and confident, the diabetic person has to become familiar with certain basic rules, which we have tried to outline above. In order to learn the basic guidelines, and how to adjust one's treatment to take part in sport, contact with a team of experienced professionals is a necessity. In addition, personal experience, together with frequent blood glucose checks, permits each person to adapt the general principles to his or her own personal situation. The national diabetes associations and the International Diabetic Athletes' Association offer publications, workshops and classes which give welcome opportunities for building up knowledge in both sport and diabetes and for sharing experiences with others.

REFERENCES

1. American Diabetes Association. Diabetes Mellitus and Exercise: Position Statement. *Diabetes Care* 1997; **20**: 1908–1912
2. Ruderman N, Devlin JT (eds) *The Health Professional's Guide to Diabetes and Exercise*. American Diabetes Association, Alexandria, 1995
3. Kang J. Robertson RJ *et al*. Effect of exercise intensity on glucose and insulin metabolism in obese individuals and obese NIDDM patients. *Diabetes Care* 1996; **19**: 341–349
4. Hagenfeldt L, Wahren J. Human forearm muscle metabolism during exercise uptake, release and oxidation of individual FFA and glycerol. *Scand. J. Clin. Lab. Invest.* 1968; **21**: 263–276
5. Lemon PWR, Nagle FJ. Effects of exercise on protein and amino acid metabolism. *Med. Sci. Sports Exerc.* 1981; **13**: 141–149
6. Koivisto VA. Diabetes and exercise. In: *The Diabetes Annual 6*. Alberti KGMM, Krall LP (eds.) Elsevier Science Publishers, Amsterdam 1991; 169–183
7. Moesch H, Décombaz J. *Nutrition et Sport*. Nestlé SA (ed.) Vevey, Switzerland, 1990
8. Wahren J, Felig P, Ahlborg G, Jorfeldt L. Glucose metabolism during leg exercise in man. *J. Clin. Invest.* 1971; **50**: 2715–2725
9. Ahlborg G, Felig P, Hagenfeld L, Hendler R, Wahren J. Substrate turnover during prolonged exercise in man. Splanchnic and leg metabolism of glucose, FFA and amino acids. *J. Clin. Invest.* 1974; **53**: 1080–1090

10. Stein TP, Hoyit RW, O'Toole M *et al*. Protein and energy metabolism during prolonged exercise in trained athletes. *Int. J. Sports Med*. 1989; **10:** 311–316

11. Wasserman DH, Lacy DB, Goldstein RE, Williams PE, Cherrington AD. Exercise-induced fall in insulin and hepatic carbohydrate metabolism during exercise. *Am. J. Physiol*. 1989; **256:** E500–508

12. Wasserman DH. Control of glucose fluxes during exercise in the absorptive state. *Annu. Rev. Physiol*. 1985; 191–218

13. Wasserman DH, Zinmann B. Fuel homeostasis. In: *The Health Professional's Guide to Diabetes and Exercise*. Ruderman N, Devlin JT (eds). American Diabetes Association, Alexandria, 1995; 27–47

14. Mitchell TH, Abraham G, Schiffrin A, Leiter LA, Marliss EB. Hyperglycaemia after intense exercise in IDDM subjects during continuous subcutaneous insulin infusion. *Diabetes Care* 1988; **11:** 311–317

15. Purdon C, Brousson M, Nyreen SL *et al*. The roles of insulin and catecholamines in the glucoregulatory response during intense exercise and early recovery in insulin-dependent diabetic and control subjects. *J. Clin. Endocrinol. Metab*. 1993; **76:** 566–573

16. Hoelzer DR, Dalsky GP, Schwartz NS *et al*. Epinephrine is not critical to prevention of hypoglycemia during exercise in humans. *Am. J. Physiol* 1986; **251:** E104–110

17. Wahrenberg H, Engfeldt P, Bolinder J, Arner P. Acute adaptation in adrenergic control of lipolysis during physical exercise in humans. *Am. J. Physiol*. 1987; **253:** E383–390

18. Zinman B. Exercise in the patient with diabetes mellitus. In: *Diabetes Mellitus*. Galloway JA. Potvin JH, Shuman CR (eds). Lilly Research Laboratories, Indianapolis, 1988, 216–223

19. Frid A, Linde B. Intraregional differences in the absorption of unmodified insulin from the abdominal wall. *Diabetic Med*. 1992; **9:** 236–239

20. Vora JP. Relationship between absorption of radiolabeled soluble insulin, subcutaneous blood flow and anthropometry. *Diabetes Care* 1992; **9:** 236–239

21. Sindelka G, Heinemann L, Berger M, Frenck W, Chantelau E. Effect of insulin concentration, subcutaneous fat thickness and skin temperature on subcutaneous insulin absorption in healthy subjects. *Diabetologia* 1994; **37:** 377–380

22. Köhlendorf K, Bojsen J, Deckert T. Absorption and miscibility of regular porcine insulin after subcutaneous injection of insulin-treated diabetic patients. *Diabetes Care* 1983; **6:** 6–9

23. Koivisto VA, Felig P. Effects of leg exercise on insulin absorption in diabetic patients. *N. Engl. J. Med*. 1978; **298:** 77–83

24. Kemmer FW, Berchtold P, Berger M *et al*. Exercise-induced fall of blood glucose in insulin-treated diabetics unrelated to alteration of insulin mobilization. *Diabetes* 1979; **28:** 1131–1137

25. Frid A, Østman J, Linde B. Hypoglycemia risk during exercise after intramuscular injection of insulin in the thigh in IDDM. *Diabetes Care* 1990; **13**: 473–477

26. Lawrence RD. The effect of exercise on insulin action in diabetes. *BMJ* 1926; **1**: 648–650

27. McDonald MJ. Post-exercise late-onset hypoglycemia in insulin-dependent diabetic patients. *Diabetes Care* 1987; **10**: 584–588

28. Sonnenberg GE, Kemmer FW, Berger M. Exercise in Type I (insulin-dependent) diabetic patients treated with continuous subcutaneous insulin infusion: prevention of exercise-induced hypoglycemia. *Diabetologia* 1990; **33**: 696–703

29. Amiel SA, Sherwin RS, Simonson DC, Tamborlane WV. Effect of intensive insulin therapy on glycemic thresholds for counterregulatory hormone release. *Diabetes* 1988; **37**: 901–907

30. Berger M, Berchtold P, Cuippers HJ *et al*. Metabolic and hormonal effects of muscular exercise in juvenile type diabetes. *Diabetologia* 1977; **13**: 355–365

31. Grimm JJ, Golay A, Habicht F, Berné C, Muchnick, S. Prevention of hypoglycemia during exercise: more carbohydrate or less insulin? *Diabetes* 1996; **45** (Suppl. 2): 104A (abstract)

32. Tuominen JA, Karonen SL, Melamies L, Bolli G, Koivisto VA. Exercise-induced hypoglycemia in IDDM patients treated with a short-acting insulin analogue. *Diabetologia* 1995; **38**: 106–111

33. Austernat E, Stahl T. *Insulinpumpentherapie*. Walter de Gruyter (eds). Berlin, New York, 1989

34. Berger W, Grimm JJ. *Praxis der intensivierten Insulintherapie*. George Thieme, Stuttgart; 1995

35. Gordon NF. *Diabetes – your complete exercise guide*. Champain, IL, Human Kinetics Publishers, 1993, 39

36. Sane T, Helve E, Pelkonen R, Koivisto VA. The adjustment of diet and insulin dose during long-term endurance exercise in Type I (insulin-dependent) diabetic men. *Diabetologia* 1988; **31**: 35–40

37. Walsh J, Roberts R, Jovanovic-Peterson, L. *Stop the Rollercoaster*. San Diego, CA, Torrey Pines Press, 1996, 141

38. Powell KE, Pratt M. Physical activity and health. *BMJ* 1996; **313**: 126–127

3

Exercise in Type 2 Diabetes

DINESH NAGI

Pinderfields Hospital, Wakefield, UK

The importance of regular physical activity in the treatment of diabetes mellitus has been realised for centuries[1], and regular physical activity has been suggested to have an important role in the management of type 2 diabetes[2,3]. Physical activity, combined with diet, was the sole form of treatment for diabetes in the pre-insulin era. Over the last two decades the potential benefits of physical activity in type 2 diabetes have become clearer, and the reasons for these benefits better understood[4]. Physical activity may also have a role in the prevention of type 2 diabetes[5], and studies to assess whether regular activity, sustained over prolonged periods of time, will prevent or delay the development of type 2 diabetes in high-risk individuals are in progress[6].

Physical activity is generally accepted as an important component of the treatment plan for type 2 diabetes because of its effects on plasma glucose concentrations. In addition, there are favourable changes in other risk factors for cardiovascular disease. These include obesity, hypertension, hyperlipidaemia and abnormalities of fibrinolysis/coagulation, which are integral parts of the 'metabolic syndrome'. Although hyperglycaemia is intimately related to the microvascular complications of diabetes, the association between hyperglycaemia and macrovascular disease is less clear[7]. No randomised trials of any treatments in type 2 diabetes have shown that good glycaemic control reduces mortality from macrovascular disease

Exercise and Sport in Diabetes. Edited by Bill Burr and Dinesh Nagi.
© 1999 John Wiley & Sons Ltd.

(which is the major cause of death in these subjects[8]). Many patients with type 2 diabetes are sedentary and may be unable to increase their physical activity levels because of either chronic complications of diabetes or associated medical conditions[9,10]. There are great problems in trying to increase the amount of regular physical activity undertaken by patients with type 2 diabetes, and to improve this state of affairs is a challenge for behaviour therapists and clinicians.

The purpose of this chapter is to assess the role of physical activity in the modern approach to diabetes management. There are no long-term studies, and therefore most of the data is from short-term, sometimes inadequately randomised, studies.

The following questions are relevant to the promotion of physical activity as a part of management strategy:

1. Does it have short- and long-term effects on glycaemic control?
2. Does it have a beneficial effect on associated risk factors such as hypertension, and dyslipidaemia?
3. Does it improve the quality of life in diabetes?
4. Does it have any effect on cardiovascular disease?
5. Does it reduce long-term mortality?
6 Are there any effects on specific complications of diabetes?
7. Is the risk/benefit ratio good enough for us to recommend it as an integral part of the treatment plan?

It is hoped that the answers will be provided in the following sections.

TYPE 2 DIABETES, INSULIN RESISTANCE AND THE METABOLIC SYNDROME

It is now generally agreed that type 2 diabetes results from a combination of insulin resistance and beta cell dysfunction[11]. However, type 2 diabetes is a heterogeneous disorder, and the relative roles of these abnormalities in its pathogenesis may vary in different populations and also among subjects within the same population[12]. There is evidence that insulin deficiency and autoimmunity may play a relatively greater role in Caucasian subjects[13,14]. The natural history of the disease suggests that increasing duration of diabetes and worsening of hyperglycaemia eventually lead to a state of beta cell failure[15]. A substantial proportion of subjects with type 2 diabetes will eventually need insulin treatment to achieve good glycaemic control and to maintain quality of life[16].

During the early twentieth century, Himsworth showed that subjects with diabetes can be broadly categorised into those who are 'insulin sensitive' (now known as type 1) and 'insulin insensitive' (type 2), based on their plasma glucose responses to an oral glucose load given with a subcutaneous insulin injection[17]. Subsequently, using sophisticated techniques, it has been shown that insulin resistance is a universal feature of type 2 diabetes[18]. Interestingly, up to 25% of non-diabetic individuals may have insulin resistance, which is quantitatively similar to that seen in subjects with type 2 diabetes[19].

Studies during the early 1960s showed that insulin resistance, hyperinsulinaemia and impaired glucose tolerance are frequently associated with coronary artery disease[20,21]. In 1985, Modan *et al.* showed an association between hypertension, glucose intolerance, obesity and hyperinsulinaemia, and proposed that insulin resistance and its consequent hyperinsulinaemia might be the pathophysiological basis[22]. Reaven drew attention to the coexistence of multiple metabolic risk factors in certain individuals, for which he coined the term 'syndrome X'. This syndrome is characterised by glucose intolerance, hyperinsulinaemia, increased VLDL-triglyceride, decreased HDL-cholesterol and hypertension[23]. Reaven proposed that insulin resistance and the consequent hyperinsulinaemia were common antecedents for this metabolic syndrome (Figure 3.1), and that these might be involved in the aetiology and clinical course of type 2 diabetes, hypertension and coronary artery disease.

Since then other variables, such as raised levels of plasminogen activator inhibitor (PAI-1) and fibrinogen, have been added to the list of features of this syndrome, which is now more commonly known as 'the metabolic syndrome'[24]. Most subjects who have features of the metabolic syndrome are obese and also have a central distribution of fat (increased waist-to-hip ratio), which is associated with insulin resistance and hyperinsulinaemia[25]. Interestingly, for the purpose of this review, physical inactivity seems to be an important component of the metabolic syndrome[26].

The association of insulin resistance, hyperinsulinaemia, central obesity and adverse cardiovascular risk factors has been shown in various studies[27,28], despite poorly understood mechanisms[29,30]. There

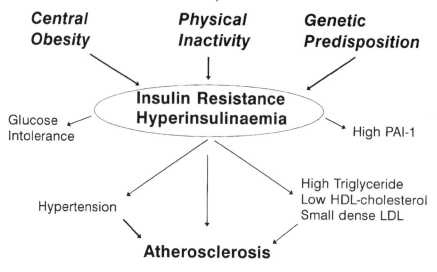

Figure 3.1. Components of the metabolic syndrome

is still considerable debate as to whether insulin resistance *per se* or its consequent hyperinsulinaemia is the proximate cause of the metabolic syndrome; epidemiological data would not favour the latter[26].

It is generally agreed that clustering of multiple risk factors in subjects with diabetes may predate the clinical diagnosis of diabetes and contribute to the excess risk of cardiovascular disease in these subjects at the time of diagnosis and thereafter[31]. Data from the San Antonio Heart Study showed higher levels of cardiovascular risk factors and hyperinsulinaemia at baseline in subjects who developed diabetes during 8-year follow up than in those who did not. The MRFIT trial showed that, in subjects with type 2 diabetes, the risk of cardiovascular death increased sharply in those who had two or more risk factors[32], confirming the earlier well known finding of increased cardiovascular mortality in subjects with diabetes observed in the Framingham data[33].

In subjects with type 2 diabetes, physical inactivity is related both to obesity and to central or abdominal fat distribution[34]. Lack of regular physical activity may contribute to the development of insulin resistance either directly or through weight gain, so that an increase in physical activity might be expected to improve the metabolic syndrome associated with insulin resistance in subjects with type 2 diabetes.

EFFECT OF EXERCISE ON THE METABOLIC SYNDROME

Work by O'Dea with Australian aborigines showed that reverting to a traditional lifestyle of 'hunting and gathering' for 7 weeks produced a marked improvement in glucose intolerance and a reduction in plasma triglyceride and blood pressure[35]. On average, fasting plasma glucose fell by 5 mmol/l and subjects lost 10 kg in weight. These changes were not due solely to increased physical activity, as their diet changed both in quality and quantity. Nevertheless, this study provided evidence that lifestyle modifications, with changes in physical activity, are likely to improve the various components of the metabolic syndrome.

The fact that the effects of exercise become apparent after a fairly short period of time and without weight loss was shown in a study by Rogers *et al.*[36] In this study, a 7-day programme of moderate intensity exercise, without any change in body weight, was associated with improved glucose tolerance and a fall in prandial insulin concentrations in subjects with type 2 diabetes. In addition to a fall in fasting and post-prandial insulin levels after exercise, there was a tendency towards an earlier insulin peak, suggesting that exercise has the potential to modify both insulin resistance and insulin secretion, two of the fundamental defects implicated in the pathogenesis of type 2 diabetes.

A study by Wing *et al.*[37], who randomised subjects with type 2 diabetes to a programme of diet alone or diet and exercise, further confirmed the possible benefits of exercise alone or combined with diet. In this study, all subjects were given similar dietary advice. Subjects in the exercise group in addition walked 3 miles a day, 3–4 times per week. Subjects were assessed over a 60-week period. The diet and exercise group lost on average twice the amount of weight lost by those randomised to diet alone over an initial 20-week period, and were able to maintain this difference at 60 weeks (Figure 3.2).

Glycaemic control improved in both groups to a similar extent, but in further analyses the magnitude of improvement in glycaemic control, as judged by glycated haemoglobin levels and the degree of weight loss, were related to the amount of physical activity (Figure 3.3).

In addition, a higher proportion of subjects in the diet and exercise group (83%) were able to reduce their drug treatment for diabetes

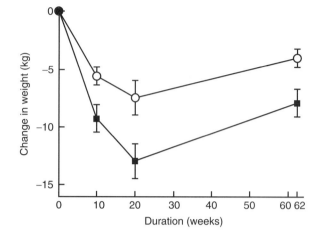

Figure 3.2. Effect of diet alone (●) or diet and exercise (■) on weight loss in subjects with type 2 diabetes Reproduced from reference 37 by permission of the author and Springer-Verlag GmbH

than in the diet-alone group (37%). Although this study had a small number of subjects, the results were extremely encouraging and showed that exercise combined with diet can lead to more weight loss, than diet alone.

A randomised study of the effects of physical training by Vanninen et al.[38] showed a significant initial decrease in body weight, fasting

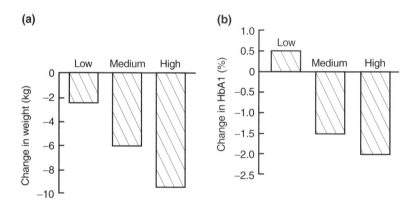

Figure 3.3. Changes in weight (a) and glycated haemoglobin (b) by physical activity level in subjects with type 2 diabetes. Reproduced from reference 37 by permission of the author and Springer-Verlag GmbH

blood glucose and glycated haemoglobin (HbA1c). They observed that physical fitness (as assessed by $\dot{V}O_2$max) was lower in subjects with type 2 diabetes. There was an inverse correlation between $\dot{V}O_2$max and HbA1c, suggesting that improvement in physical fitness may be associated with better glycaemic control. Over a longer time period, improvement was observed only in female subjects, although some fall in glucose and insulin levels was noted at one year in most subjects[38].

A recent study by Larsen *et al.* analysed the effects of moderate exercise on post-prandial glucose homeostasis[39]. They showed a beneficial effect of exercise on glycaemia and insulin levels, but the effect persisted only in the post-absorptive phase of that meal and not the following meal. They also found that a reduction in the calorie content of the meal, equivalent to the energy expended during exercise, had the same effect. The practical implications are that a patient with diabetes could choose to eat *ad libitum* and subsequently expend these calories by exercise. While this approach may be useful for lean subjects, it would hardly be of practical value in obese subjects with type 2 diabetes, for whom weight reduction is the main aim and some sort of calorie restriction is essential.

A study by Lehmann *et al.* showed that a regular aerobic exercise programme at 50–70% maximal effort for 3 months led to a 20% reduction in fasting plasma triglyceride concentrations and an increase in HDL-lipoprotein subfraction[40]. In this study there was a significant reduction in systolic and diastolic blood pressure—and, more importantly, a significant fall in waist-to-hip ratio—which were independent of body weight and glycaemic control. There were no significant changes in glycaemic control in the intervention group, although in the control group HbA1c rose by 0.6%. These studies all showed clear-cut benefits but were short-term studies. Further evidence is needed to confirm that adherence to exercise can be maintained over a longer period and that the benefits observed in short-term studies can be maintained.

A study by Eriksson and Lindgarde[41] showed that an outpatient exercise programme could be maintained successfully for up to 6 years. This was a non-randomised study of primary prevention of type 2 diabetes, which involved 41 patients with known type 2 diabetes and 161 subjects with impaired glucose tolerance (IGT). There was a significant improvement in glucose tolerance and post-prandial insulin concentrations despite a fairly modest amount of weight loss. In 28% of subjects with diabetes the glucose tolerance had returned to normal, 26% of subjects reverted to IGT and 46% were still classified as diabetic. In subjects who had IGT at baseline, 69% had normal glucose tolerance and 21% still had IGT; 11% had developed diabetes, compared with 21% in the control group. The most valid and encouraging conclusion of this study was that an outpatient-based exercise programme could be successfully maintained for up to 5 years. Barnard *et al.* also showed that the effect of exercise on fasting plasma glucose was related to pharmacological treatment of diabetes and was larger in those on diet alone than in those on oral hypogly-caemic or insulin treatment[42]. This observation would suggest that exercise is likely to be most beneficial early in the course of the disease.

Overall compliance with outpatient-based exercise programmes remains poor[9, 10]. In a study by Schneider *et al.*[10], compliance dropped to 20% by the end of 12 months. As in the above studies, subjects who took part in this programme of diet and exercise showed significant weight loss, lower fasting plasma glucose and lower fasting plasma triglyceride levels at 3 months which were maintained for up to 1 year. Key observations in this study are worth reviewing: first, the best predictors of long-term compliance were self-referral, participa-tion of spouse, and female sex; secondly, even those subjects who dropped out of the programme at 3 months were taking some sort of physical activity when interviewed a year later. In the study by Wing *et al.* compliance with exercise, as judged by calories expended, was excellent for the duration of the study even though after 20 weeks subjects were left to do their walking by themselves[37]. It seems that an initial intensive training period may improve long-term compliance, so that formal programmes may best be used for initial patient education to prepare individuals to exercise safely and appropriately on their own, choosing activities which fit into their daily lifestyle.

EFFECTS ON CARDIOVASCULAR RISK FACTORS

Most of the studies discussed above have also shown beneficial effects on lipids and blood pressure. The study by Rogers *et al.*[36] showed a fall in systolic blood pressure of 6 mmHg and a 33% reduction in plasma triglyceride concentrations. Wing *et al.* showed a significant reduction in serum cholesterol and plasma triglyceride concentrations, which was significant at 10 weeks but not at one year[37]. HDL-cholesterol levels remained higher after one year of follow-up but no changes were observed in systolic and diastolic blood pressures. Schneider *et al.*, in their study, showed improvements of approximately 25% in plasma triglycerides but no change in LDL-cholesterol[43]. Similar beneficial effects were maintained in the Malmo study for up to 6 years. Krotkiewsky *et al.* noticed that the best response occurred in subjects who had the highest baseline fasting insulin concentration[44], a finding confirmed by Schneider *et al*[43]. These findings would suggest that the mechanisms for changes in lipids following exercise are intimately related to changes in insulin resistance.

Increased physical activity is associated with a fall in plasma triglyceride and a rise in HDL-cholesterol[45,46]. The effect on LDL-cholesterol concentration is only modest but there may be beneficial effects on the composition of LDL particles. It would also appear that, to gain maximum benefits in terms of improvements in lipids, moderate-intensity exercise might be required. For instance, in non-diabetic subjects the effects on lipids increased with increasing exercise in a dose-dependent manner up to a distance of 40 miles/week[47]. Insulin resistance is universally associated with high plasma triglyceride and low HDL-cholesterol concentration[48]. Impaired lipoprotein lipase (LPL) activity is usually associated with insulin resistance states and exercise is likely to achieve beneficial effects on plasma triglyceride and HDL-cholesterol by influencing both muscle and hepatic LPL activity[45]. Change in the former will lead to a greater extraction and clearance of VLDL at the periphery and in the latter to reduced release of VLDL into the circulation from the liver. Other possible mechanisms, such as enhanced reverse cholesterol transport, may also be important. Some of the effects of exercise on lipids may be indirect and related to loss of abdominal fat. As a consequence, there would be less mobilisation of FFA from abdominal fat to liver, and reduced hepatic VLDL production[49].

Essential hypertension has been intimately linked to insulin resistance[50]. One mechanism by which hyperinsulinaemia is related to blood pressure in type 2 diabetes is through its effects on the sympathetic nervous system and renal sodium handling[51,52]. A reduction in blood pressure following increase in physical activity is significantly related to improvement in insulin sensitivity, correlated with reduced fasting hyperinsulinaemia and independent of change in weight[53]. Regular physical activity may lower blood pressure, on average, by 8–10 mmHg. Improvements in blood pressure of this magnitude, if sustained, have the potential significantly to lower cerebrovascular, and possibly cardiovascular, mortality.

There are data to suggest that regular physical activity might have beneficial effects on fibrinolysis, although the results remain somewhat inconsistent. Schneider *et al.* showed improved fibrinolysis following 6 weeks of exercise in subjects with type 2 diabetes[54]. Gris *et al.* showed similar benefits, and these were associated with lower levels of PAI-1[55]. PAI-1 has been shown to be related to insulin resistance, and the lowering of PAI-1 and fibrinolysis is also related to improvements in circulating insulin and plasma triglyceride concentrations, both of which are related to insulin resistance[56]. There are no long-term studies of the effects of exercise on fibrinolysis. As raised levels of PAI-1 are shown to predict recurrence of acute myocardial infarction in non-diabetic and diabetic subjects[57,58], it is possible that the effects of exercise in lowering PAI-1 and plasma fibrinogen levels may produce long-term reduction in cardiovascular events.

REGULATION OF CARBOHYDRATE METABOLISM DURING EXERCISE

The effects of exercise on carbohydrate metabolism are discussed in detail in Chapter 1. During exercise, there is a strong negative relationship between plasma glucose concentration and hepatic glucose production. In subjects with type 2 diabetes, the regulation of carbohydrate metabolism during and immediately after exercise may differ from that in non-diabetic subjects. Hepatic glucose production during exercise is generally reduced in type 2 diabetes and the strong negative relationship between plasma glucose and hepatic glucose output seen in non-diabetic subjects is generally lacking. This would suggest that the feedback control of glucose production from the liver by plasma glucose is impaired in diabetes[59]. A study by Kjaer *et al.* showed that, 10 min after an acute bout of exercise, the observed rise in plasma glucose was higher in type 2 diabetes due to uninhibited and excess hepatic glucose production. This initial rise in plasma glucose due to exaggerated counter-regulatory hormone responses is followed by a period during which insulin sensitivity seems to continue to improve for up to 24 h[60]. A study by Schneider *et al.*[61] showed that after 6 weeks of physical training there was a blunting of the exercise-induced increase in counter-regulatory hormones in non-diabetic but not in diabetic subjects. Exercise resulted in a decrease in plasma glucose in subjects with diabetes 30 min after exercise but an increase in non-diabetic subjects.

From these studies it is clear that maximum dynamic exercise in subjects with type 2 diabetes, because of exaggerated counter regulatory responses, results in a short period of hyperglycaemia and hyperinsulinaemia. However, this is followed by a period of 'insulin sensitisation' with a beneficial effect on glucose utilisation. In summary, glucose turnover after exercise in type 2 diabetes is heterogeneous and may show a fall, a sustained rise or no change. These differences are likely to be due to impaired non-pancreatic hormonal responses[60,61].

EFFECT OF EXERCISE ON INSULIN SENSITIVITY

The earliest indication that exercise has the potential to improve insulin sensitivity was put forward by Bjorntorp[62]. After 12 weeks of exercise or physical training, subjects showed a substantial fall in circulating fasting and post-prandial insulin concentrations without any change in plasma glucose levels[63]. Subsequently, Rosenthal *et al.* showed that insulin sensitivity was directly related to physical training as measured by $\dot{V}O_2$max, both in men and in women[64]. Studies using the hyperinsulinaemic clamp showed that insulin-stimulated glucose uptake increased following a single bout of physical training[59,65]. This improvement in insulin sensitivity is confined to exercising muscles and is partly due to replenishment of the glycogen stores that were depleted during exercise, while non-exercising muscles are relatively insulin resistant immediately following exercise[66,67].

The mechanism of glucose disposal may differ between subjects with type 2 diabetes who are treated with dietary modification alone and those with diet and exercise[68]. In this study, subjects who exercised in addition to changing their diet mainly used the non-oxidative (glycogen synthesis) route for glucose disposal, while those on diet alone used oxidative pathways (glucose oxidation). These observations provide a pathophysiological basis for an additive effect of diet and exercise on insulin sensitivity. Devlin *et al.* showed similar results in subjects with type 2 diabetes (i.e. the effect of exercise was on non-oxidative glucose disposal)[64]. After a single bout of exercise in subjects with type 2 diabetes, both peripheral and hepatic insulin sensitivity improved (Figure 3.4). They also found lower basal hepatic glucose output after exercise, which was accompanied by lower fasting plasma glucose on the morning after the exercise[65].

There is still no universal agreement as to the intensity and duration of exercise needed to improve insulin sensitivity. Most studies suggest that exercise intensity of at least 40–50% $\dot{V}O_2$max (which is considered to be of moderate intensity) is needed to improve insulin sensitivity[69]. Exercise of this intensity is associated with some glycogen depletion,

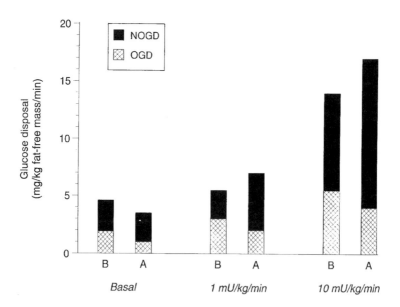

Figure 3.4. Effect of exercise on oxidative (OGD; ▨) and non-oxidative glucose disposal (NODG ■) at baseline and during low-dose (1 mU/kg/min) and high-dose (10 mU/kg/min) hyperinsulinameic euglycaemic clamp studies in subjects with type 2 diabetes. B = before exercise; A = after exercise Reproduced by permission from ref. 66

which may be a prerequisite for enhancing glucose disposal following exercise[65]. The underlying cellular mechanisms by which these beneficial effects occur are not fully elucidated. Studies have shown that exercise improves the number of insulin receptors[70] as well as tissue levels of glucose transporters (GLUT 4), thereby facilitating glucose transport into the cells and its disposal through insulin-sensitive pathways[71].

The improvement in insulin sensitivity following a single bout of exercise has been shown to last for up to 60 h, and is completely normalised to pre-exercise levels by 3–5 days[72]. Repeated bouts of moderate intensity exercise may, however, provide adaptive mechanisms, which are associated with a long-term increase in insulin sensitivity[73,74]. From a practical point of view, it seems likely that a modest fall in plasma glucose levels following repeated bouts of physical activity at intervals not longer than 48–60 h may be associated with long-term changes in glycaemic control.

To summarise, regular physical activity in subjects with type 2 diabetes is associated with improved short-term, and probably long-term, glycaemic control. In addition, there are beneficial changes in associated cardiovascular risk factors such as blood pressure, dyslipidaemia and abnormalities of thrombosis and coagulation. These changes appear to be intimately related to beneficial changes in insulin sensitivity and appear to be most obvious around the time of diagnosis and early in the course of the disease. In addition, regular physical activity when combined with dietary modification leads to more profound weight loss and may help in long-term weight maintenance.

EXERCISE AND PREVENTION OF TYPE 2 DIABETES

The prevalence of diabetes is rising rapidly world-wide, and certain developing nations are currently experiencing a rise in the prevalence of type 2 diabetes of epidemic proportions[75]. This is likely to have huge socioeconomic consequences in these countries due to the costs associated with the complications of type 2 diabetes[76]. Primary prevention of type 2 diabetes is therefore of particular interest to health economists.

Type 2 diabetes has a number of disease characteristics, which make it potentially preventable[5,77]. Considerable knowledge exists about the risk factors for diabetes which are potentially modifiable[78]. There is a strong genetic predisposition to the disease and environmental factors play an important role in the development of clinical diabetes. In most subjects predisposed to develop type 2 diabetes, there is a long period during which minor degrees of glucose intolerance exist[78-82]: this stage of pre-diabetes can be recognised by performing an oral glucose tolerance test and is known as 'impaired glucose tolerance' (IGT). Measuring fasting plasma glucose identifies a state known as impaired fasting glucose (IFG)[83,84]. Subjects thus identified are at a higher risk of diabetes than those whose glucose tolerance is normal[79-82]. Identification of subjects at high risk of diabetes provides us with an opportunity to modify the disease process, to either delay it or prevent it manifesting clinically.

Both insulin resistance and defective insulin secretion contribute to the development of diabetes[11,12,18], and both are modifiable through lifestyle interventions and/or pharmacological therapy[5]. In spite of this, it has only recently been shown that type 2 diabetes can be prevented[85].

Although there are a number of strategies for disease prevention, behaviour modification through diet and exercise is attractive and has the added advantage of modifying other associated conditions such as coronary artery disease, hypertension and obesity[86]. Lifestyle modifications are extremely difficult to sustain over the lifetime of an individual. It is likely that different strategies may need to be adopted in different ethnic groups to improve adherence to measures which promote healthy lifestyles[87].

A number of observational studies (Table 3.1) have shown that regular physical activity has a protective effect on the development of type 2 diabetes. These studies were remarkable for their consistent findings for the protective effects of physical activity on the occurrence of type 2 diabetes. Some of the studies also showed a dose–response relationship between the frequency of physical activity and the degree of protective effect[88-92]. These studies suggest a causative role for physical inactivity in type 2 diabetes.

In the Physician Health Study published by Manson *et al.*[88], 21,271 males were followed over a 5-year period. The incidence of diabetes was negatively related to frequency of exercise (369 cases per 100,000

Table 3.1. Prospective studies of physical activity and risk of type 2 diabetes

Study population	Reference	Follow-up	Sex	Protective effect of exercise
US College Alumni	89	Variable	Female	Yes
Pennsylvania Alumni	93	14 years	Male	Yes
Nurses' Health Study	90	8 years	Female	Yes
Malmo Study	41	6 years	Male	Yes
Physician Health Study	88	5 years	Male	Yes

person-years in those who exercised less than once a week and 214 in those who exercised more than five times per week). The age-adjusted risk of diabetes in men who exercised at least once a week was 0.64 compared with those who exercised less frequently.

In the study by Helmrich *et al.*[89], type 2 diabetes was observed in 202 out of 5990 male subjects. In this study, leisure-time physical activity, expressed as number of calories expended, was found to be inversely related to the development of diabetes. The age-adjusted risk of diabetes was 6% lower for each 500 kilocalories expended. The beneficial effects of exercise remained significant when adjusted for the confounding effects of obesity, parental history of diabetes and blood pressure.

In the Nurses Health Study[90], women who participated in vigorous physical activity at least once a week had a risk of diabetes which was 33% lower than that in those who did not take part in such activity. No dose–response relationship between frequency of exercise and risk of diabetes was seen in this study.

In the Honolulu Heart Study[91], subjects were followed for 6 years and the cumulative incidence of diabetes was lower with increasing levels of physical activity in both men and women. The age-adjusted odds ratio for diabetes, comparing subjects who were in the upper quintile with those in the lower four quintiles, was 0.55 in men and 0.50 in women.

A study of 897 middle-aged Finnish men (recently published by Lynch *et al.*[92]) showed that self-reported moderate-intensity exercise undertaken for 40 min/week was associated with a 56% lower risk of type 2 diabetes. They also found that high levels of cardiorespiratory physical fitness (oxygen consumption in a respiratory chamber) also

Exercise and Sport in Diabetes

had a protective effect on the development of diabetes. In subjects at high risk of diabetes who took a moderate degree of physical activity for more than 40 min once a week the risk of diabetes was 64% lower than in those who did not take any physical activity.

All the above studies were observational cohort studies and indicate the need for well designed, randomised clinical trials to assess the effects of interventions incorporating physical activity on the future development of type 2 diabetes.

There have been very few studies of the effect of exercise intervention on preventing type 2 diabetes. The study by Eriksson *et al.*, mentioned earlier[41], showed that it is possible for subjects to comply with a behaviour modification for up to six years. No other conclusions can be drawn because the study was not randomised and had a relatively small number of subjects.

The Da-Qing study from China[85] was a population-based randomised study. A total of 576 subjects with IGT were randomised to four groups (control, diet alone, exercise alone or both). They were followed for a period of 5.6 years and the incidence of diabetes was reduced in all three groups (Table 3.2).

Some general points of interest emerged from this first properly randomised and controlled intervention study:

- Lifestyle interventions in the form of diet and physical activity for up to 6 years significantly reduced the development of diabetes.
- The effects of diet and exercise were similar—both reduced the risk of diabetes.
- The risk of diabetes was reduced despite fairly modest reductions in body weight (approximately 2 kg).
- The effects were similar in obese and non-obese subjects.

Table 3.2. The Da-Qing study from China

Intervention	Cumulative incidence %
Control group	67
Diet only	44
Exercise only	41
Diet and exercise	46

From reference 85, by permission

- The increase in physical activity was modest but was sustained over the period of the study.

These results clearly need to be replicated in other racial groups; in particular those with a high risk of type 2 diabetes. A large multi-centre study (Diabetes Prevention Project) is currently under way in the USA, and aims to recruit 4000 subjects at high risk of type 2 diabetes. Eligibility criteria include age over 25 years, minimal degree of overweight, and IGT as defined by WHO criteria. This study will include 50% women, up to 50% of subjects will be non-Caucasian and 25% will be over 65 years old. Intensive lifestyle interventions will be tested, along with pharmacological interventions to modify insulin resistance. The results of this study should be available in the year 2002 and will provide evidence not only as to the possibility of preventing type 2 diabetes, but also on the relative effects of lifestyle modifications and pharmacological interventions[6].

It is now well established that IGT and IFG are risk factors for future development of diabetes, macrovascular disease, hypertension and dyslipidaemia. While we await the result of the Diabetes Prevention Project, it will be reasonable for us to advise these at-risk subjects, as well as those with type 2 diabetes, to follow a healthy lifestyle, which should include regular physical activity. At the same time we should take an aggressive approach in treating hypertension, dyslipidaemia, obesity and smoking.

REFERENCES

1. Sushruta SCS. *Vaidya Jadavaji Trikamji Acharia* 13th Rev, 3rd Ed. Bombay: Nirnyar Sagar Press, 1938 (original book published in 500 BC)
2. American Diabetes Association. Exercise and NIDDM (Technical Review). *Diabetes Care* 1990; **13:** 785–789
3. American Diabetes Association. Diabetes mellitus and exercise (Position Statement). *Diabetes Care* 1990; **13:** 804–805
4. Schneider SH, Morgado A. Effects of fitness and physical training on carbohydrate metabolism and associated cardiovascular risk factors in patients with diabetes. *Diabetes Rev* 1995; **3:** 378–407
5. Knowler WC, Narayan KMV, Hanson RL *et al.* Perspective in Diabetes. Preventing Non-insulin-dependent Diabetes. *Diabetes* 1995; **44:** 483–488

6. National Institutes of Health. Non-insulin Dependent Diabetes Primary Prevention Trial. *NIH Guide Grants Contacts* 1993; **22:** 1–20
7. Barrett-Connor E. Does hyperglycaemia really cause coronary artery disease? *Diabetes Care* 1997; **20:** 1620–1623
8. Panzram G. Mortality and survival in type 2 (non-insulin-dependent) diabetes mellitus. *Diabetologia* 1987; **30:** 123–131
9. Samaras K, Ashwell S, Mackintosh A-M, Campbell LV, Chisholm DJ. Exercise in NIDDM: Are we Missing the Point?. *Diabetic Med* 1996; **13:** 780–781
10. Schneider SH, Khanchadurian AK, Amorosa LF, Clemow L, Ruderman NB. Ten-year experience with an exercise-based outpatient life-style modification program in the treatment of diabetes mellitus. *Diabetes Care* 1992; **15**(Suppl. 4): 1800–1810
11. DeFronzo RA. Pathogenesis of type 2 (non-insulin-dependent) diabetes mellitus: a balanced overview. *Diabetologia* 1992; **35:** 389–397
12. Turner RC, Holman RR, Matthews DR, Peto J. Relative contributions of insulin deficiency and insulin resistance in maturity-onset diabetes. *Lancet* 1982; **i:** 596–598
13. Temple RC, Carrington CA, Luzio SD *et al.* Insulin deficiency in non-insulin-dependent diabetes. *Lancet* 1989; **i:** 293-295
14. Groop L, Miettinen A, Groop PH, Meri S, Koskimies S, Bottazzo GF. Organ-specific autoimmunity and HLA-DR antigen as markers for β-cell destruction in patients with type 2 diabetes. *Diabetes* 1988; **37:** 99–103
15. DeFronzo RA. The Triumvirate: β-cell, Muscle, Liver – a collusion responsible for NIDDM. *Diabetes* 1988; **37:** 667–687
16. DeFronzo RA, Ferrannini E, Koivisto V. New concepts in the pathogenesis and treatment of non-insulin dependent diabetes mellitus. *Am J Med* 1983; **74:** 52–81
17. Himsworth H. Diabetes Mellitus: a differentiation into insulin sensitive and insulin insensitive types. *Lancet* 1936; **i:** 127–130
18. Gerich JE. Role of insulin resistance in the pathogenesis of type 2 (non-insulin-dependent) diabetes mellitus. *Clin Endocrinol Metab* 1988; **2:** 307–326
19. Hollenbeck C, Reaven GM. Variations in insulin-stimulated glucose uptake in healthy individuals with normal glucose tolerance. *J Clin Endocrinol Metab* 1987; **64:** 1169–1173
20. Welborn TA, Breckenridge A, Rubinstein AH, Dollery CT, Fraser TR. Serum insulin in essential hypertension and peripheral vascular disease. *Lancet* 1969; **i:** 1078–1080
21. Nikkila EA, Miettinen TA, Vesene M-R, Pelkonen R. Plasma insulin in coronary artery disease. *Lancet* 1965; **ii:** 508–511
22. Modan M, Halkin H, Almog S *et al.* Hyperinsulinemia: a link between

hypertension, obesity and glucose intolerance. *J Clin Invest* 1985; **75:** 809–817

23. Reaven GM. Role of insulin resistance in human disease. *Diabetes* 1988; **37:** 1595–1607

24. Landin K, Tenghorn L, Smith U. Elevated fibrinogen and plasminogen activator inhibitor (PAI-1) in hypertension are related to metabolic risk factors for cardiovascular disease. *J Intern Med* 1990; **227:** 273–278.

25. Pouliot M-C, Despres J-P, Nadeau A *et al.* Visceral obesity in man. Associations with glucose tolerance, plasma insulin, and lipoprotein levels. *Diabetes* 1992; **41:** 826–834

26. Zimmet PZ. Hyperinsulinemia – how innocent a bystander? *Diabetes Care* 1993; **16:** 56–70

27. DeFronzo RA, Ferrannini E. Insulin Resistance: A multifaceted syndrome responsible for NIDDM, obesity, hypertension, dyslipidaemia and atherosclerotic vascular disease. *Diabetes Care* 1991; **14:** 173–194

28. Haffner SM, Valdez RA, Hazuda HP, Mitchell BD, Morales PA, Stern MP. Prospective analysis of the insulin resistance syndrome (syndrome X). *Diabetes* 1992; **41:** 715–722

29. Stern MP. Diabetes and cardiovascular disease: The 'Common Soil' Hypothesis. *Diabetes* 1995; **44:** 369–374

30. Kissebah AH, Vydelingum N, Murray R *et al.* Relation of body fat distribution to metabolic complications of obesity. *J Clin Endocrinol Metab* 1982; **54:** 254–260

31. Haffner SM, Stern MP, Hazuda HP, Mitchell BD, Patterson JK. Cardiovascular risk factors in confirmed prediabetic individuals. Does the clock for coronary heart disease start ticking before the onset of clinical diabetes? *JAMA* 1990; **263:** 2893–2898

32. Stamler J, Vaccaro O, Neaton JD, Wentworth D. Diabetes, other risk factors, mortality for men screened in the Multiple Risk Factor Intervention Trial. *Diabetes Care* 1993; **16:** 434–444

33. Garcia MJ, McNamara PM, Gordon T, Kannel WB. Morbidity and mortality in diabetics in the Framingham population. Sixteen year follow-up study. *Diabetes* 1974; **23:** 105–111

34. Kriska AM, LaPorte RE. The association of physical activity with obesity, fat distribution and glucose intolerance in Pima Indians. *Diabetologia* 1993; **36:** 863–869

35. O'Dea K. Marked improvement in carbohydrate and lipid metabolism in diabetes Australian Aborigines after temporary reversion to a traditional lifestyle. *Diabetes* 1984; **33:** 596–603

36. Rogers MA, Yamamoto C, King DS, Hagberg JM, Ehasani AA, Holloszy JO. Improvement in glucose tolerance after 1 week of exercise in patients with mild NIDDM. *Diabetes Care* 1988; **11:** 613–618

37. Wing RR, Epstein LH, Paternostro-Bayles M, Kriska A, Nowalk MP, Gooding W. Exercise in a behavioral weight control programme for obese patients with type II diabetes. *Diabetologia* 1988; **31:** 902–909
38. Vanninen E, Uusitupa M, Siitonen O, Laitinen J, Lansimies E. Habitual physical activity, aerobic capacity and metabolic control in patients with newly diagnosed type II diabetes mellitus: effect of a one year diet and exercise intervention. *Diabetologia* 1992; **35:** 340–346
39. Larsen JJS, Dela F, Kjaer M, Galbo H. The effect of moderate exercise on post prandial glucose homeostasis in NIDDM patients. *Diabetologia* 1997; **40:** 447–453
40. Lehmann R, Vokac A, Niedermann K, Agosti K, Spinas GA. Loss of abdominal fat and improvement of the cardiovascular risk profile by regular moderate exercise training in patients with NIDDM. *Diabetologia* 1995; **38:** 1313–1319
41. Eriksson KF, Lindgarde F. Prevention of type 2 (non-insulin dependent) diabetes mellitus by diet and physical exercise: the six year Malmo feasibility study. *Diabetologia* 1991; **34:** 891–898
42. Barnard J, Tiffany J, Inkeles SB. Diet and exercise in the treatment of NIDDM. *Diabetes Care* 1994; **17:** 1469–1472
43. Schneider SH, Amorosa LF, Khachadurian AK, Ruderman NB. Studies on the mechanism of improved glucose control during regular exercise in type 2 (non-insulin dependent) diabetes mellitus. *Diabetologia* 1984; **26:** 355–360
44. Krotkiewski M, Loaroth P, Manrwoukas K *et al.* Effects of physical training on insulin secretion and effectiveness and glucose metabolism in obesity and type 2 diabetes mellitus. *Diabetologia* 1995; **28:** 881–890
45. Krotkiewski M, Manrwoukas K, Sjostrom L, SuDivan L, Wetterquist H, Bjorntorp P. Effects of long term physical training on body fat, metabolism and BP in obesity. *Metabolism* 1979; **28:** 650–658
46. Vu Tran, Weltman A, Glazes G, Mood D. The effects of exercise on plasma lipids and lipoproteins: a meta-analysis of studies. *Med Sci Sports Exerc* 1983; **15:** 393–402
47. Superko HR. Exercise training, serum lipids, and lipoprotein particle: is there a change threshold. *Med Sci Sports Exerc* 1991; **23:** 677–685
48. Laws A, Reaven GM. Evidence for an independent relationship between insulin resistance and fasting plasma HDL-cholesterol, triglyceride and insulin concentrations. *J Intern Med* 1992; **232:** 25–30
49. Van Gaal L, Rillaerts E, Greten W, DeLeeuw I. Relationship of body fat distribution to atherogenic risk in NIDDM. *Diabetes Care* 1988; **11:** 103–106
50. Ferrannini E, Buzzigoli G, Bonadonna R *et al.* Insulin resistance in essential hypertension. *N Engl J Med* 1987; **317:** 350–357

51. DeFronzo RA. The effect of insulin on renal sodium metabolism. *Diabetologia* 1981; **21:** 165–171
52. Landsberg L. Diet, obesity and hypertension; an hypothesis involving insulin, the sympathetic nervous system, and adaptive thermogenesis. *Q J Med* 1986; **236:** 1081–1090
53. Rocchini AP, Katch V, Schork A, Kelch RP. Insulin and blood pressure during weight loss in obese adolescents. *Hypertension* 1987; **10:** 267–273
54. Schneider SH, Kim HC, Khachandurian AK, Ruderman NB. Impaired fibrinolytic response to exercise in type 2 diabetes: effects of exercise and physical training. *Metabolism* 1988; **37:** 924–929
55. Gris JC, Schved JF, Aguilar-Martinez P, Amaud A, Sanchez N. Impact of physical training on plasminogen activator inhibitor activity in sedentary men. *Fibrinolysis* 1988; **4**(Suppl. 2): 97–98
56. Juhan Vague I, Alessi MC, Vague P. Increased plasminogen activator inhibitor 1 levels. A possible link between insulin resistance and atherothrombosis. *Diabetologia* 1991; **34:** 457–462
57. Hamsten A, Wiman B, de Faire U, Blombäck M. Increased plasma levels of a rapid inhibitor of tissue plasminogen activator in young survivors of myocardial infarction. *N Engl J Med* 1985; **313:** 1557–1563
58. Gray R, Yudkin JS, Patterson D. Plasminogen activator inhibitor: a risk factors for acute myocardial infarction in diabetic patients. *Br Heart J* 1993; **69:** 228–232
59. Jenkins AB, Furler SM, Bruce DG, Chisholm DJ. Regulation of hepatic glucose output during moderate exercise in Non-insulin dependent diabetes. *Metabolism* 1988; **10:** 966–972
60. Kjaer M, Hollenbeck CB, Frey-Hewitt B, Galbo H, Haskell W, Reaven GM. Glucoregulation and hormonal responses to maximal exercise in non-insulin dependent diabetes. *J Appl Physiol* 1990; **68:** 2067–2074
61. Schneider SH, Khachadurian AK, Amoroso LF, Gavras SE, Fineberg SE, Ruderman NB. Abnormal glucoregulation during exercise in type 2 (Non-Insulin-Dependent) diabetes. *Metabolism* 1986; **36:** 1161–1166
62. Bjorntorp P. Effects of exercise on plasma insulin. *Int J Sports Med* 1981; **2:** 125–129
63. Bjorntorp P, DeJounge K, Sjostrom L, Sullivan L. The effects of physical training on insulin production in obesity. *Metabolism* 1980; **19:** 631–638
64. Rosenthal M, Haskell WL, Solomon R, Widstrom A, Reaven GM. Demonstration of a relationship between level of physical training and insulin-stimulated glucose ultilization in normal humans. *Diabetes* 1983; **32:** 408–411
65. Devlin JT, Hirshman M, Horton ED, Horton ES. Enhanced peripheral and splanchnic insulin sensitivity in NIDDM men after a single bout of exercise. *Diabetes* 1987; **36:** 434–439

66. Horton ES, Devlin JT. Exercise and non-insulin dependent diabetes mellitus. In Current Trends in non-insulin dependent diabetes mellitus. Ed. Alberti KGMM and Mazze RS. *Excerpta Medica*, Amsterdam. 1989; 271–284

67. Ivy JL, Holloszy JO. Persistent increase in glucose uptake by rat skeletal muscle following exercise. *Am J Physiol* 1981; **241:** C200–C203

68. Bogardus C, Ravussin E, Robbins DC, Wolfe DC, Horton ES, Sims EAH. Effects of physical training and diet therapy on carbohydrate metabolism in patients with glucose intolerance and non-insulin dependent diabetes mellitus. *Diabetes* 1984; **33:** 311–318

69. King AC, Haskell Wl, Taylor CB, Kraemer HC, Debusk RF. Home based exercise training in healthy older men and women. *JAMA* 1991; **266:** 1535–1542

70. Koivisto VA, Soman V, Conrad P, Hendler R, Nadel E, Felig P. Insulin binding to monocytes in trained athletes: changes in the resting state and after exercise. *J Clin Invest* 1979; **64:** 1011–1015

71. Dohm GL, Sinha MK, Caro JF. Insulin receptor binding and protein kinase activity in muscles of trained rats. *Am J Physiol* 1987; **252:** E170–E175

72. Burnstein R, Polychronakos C, Toews CJ, MacDougall JD, Guyda HJ, Posner BI. Acute reversal of enhanced insulin action in trained athletes. *Diabetes* 1987; **36:** 434–439

73. Henriksson J. Influence of exercise on insulin sensitivity. *J Cardiovasc Risk* 1995; **2:** 303–309

74. Koivisto VA, DeFronzo RA. Exercise in the treatment of type 2 Diabetes. *Acta Endocrinol* 1984; **262:** 107–111

75. Amos AF, McCarty DJ, Zimmet P. The rising global burden of diabetes and its complications: Estimates and projections to the year 2010. *Diabetic Med* 1997; **12**(Suppl. 5): S7–S15

76. Greener M. Counting the Cost of diabetes. *Costs and Options in Diabetes* 1997; **10:** 4–5

77. Tuommilehto J, Knowler WC, Zimmet P. Primary Prevention of Non-insulin-dependent Diabetes. *Diabetes Metab Rev* 1992; **8:** 339–353

78. Bennett PH. Impaired Glucose Tolerance – a target for intervention? *Arteriosclerosis* 1985; **5:** 315–317

79. Nagi DK, Knowler WC, Charles MA *et al.* Early and late insulin response as predictors of NIDDM in Pima Indians with impaired glucose tolerance. *Diabetologia* 1995; **38:** 187–192

80. Saad MF, Knowler WC, Pettitt DJ, Nelson RG, Mott DG, Bennett PH. The natural history of glucose intolerance in the Pima Indians. *N Engl J Med* 1988; **319:** 1500–1506

81. Kadowaki T, Miyaki Y, Hagura R et al. Risk factors for worsening to diabetes in subjects with impaired glucose tolerance. *Diabetologia* 1984; **26:** 44–49

82. King H, Zimmet P, Raper LR, Balkau B. The natural history of impaired glucose tolerance in the micronesian population of Nauru: a 6 year follow-up study. *Diabetologia* 1984; **26:** 39–43

83. World Health Organization. *Diabetes Mellitus: Report of a WHO Study Group.* Technical Report Series No 727, WHO, Geneva 1985

84. Report of the expert committee on the diagnosis and classification of diabetes mellitus. *Diabetes Care* 1998; **21** (Suppl. 1) S5–S19

85. Pan X, Li G, Hu Y *et al.* Effects of diet and exercise in preventing NIDDM in people with Impaired Glucose Tolerance. *Diabetes Care* 1997; **20:** 537–544

86. King H, Kriska AM. Prevention of type 2 diabetes by physical training. *Diabetes Care* 1992; **15:** 1794–1799

87. Narayan KMV, Hoskin M, Kozak D *et al.* Randomised clinical trial of life style interventions in Pima Indians a pilot study. *Diabetic Med* 1998; **15:** 66–72

88. Manson JE, Rimm RB, Stamfer MJ *et al.* A prospective study of exercise and incidence of diabetes among US male physicians. *JAMA* 1992; **268:** 63–67

89. Helmrich SP, Ragland DR, Leung RW, Paffenbarger RS. Physical activity and reduced occurrence of non-insulin-dependent diabetes mellitus. *N Engl J Med* 1991; **325:** 147–152

90. Manson JE, Rimm RB, Stamfer MJ *et al.* Physical activity and incidence of non-insulin-dependent diabetes in women. *Lancet* 1991; **338:** 774–778

91. Burchfield CM, Sharp DS, Curb D *et al.* Physical activity and incidence of diabetes: The Honolulu Heart program. *Am J Epidemiol* 1995; **141:** 360–368

92. Lynch J, Helmrich Sp, Lokka TA *et al.* Moderately intense physical activity and high levels of cardiorespiratory fitness reduce the risk of Non-insulin dependent diabetes mellitus in middle-aged men. *Arch Intern Med* 1996; **156:** 1307–1314

93. Frisch RE, Wyshak G, Albright TE, Albright NL, Schiff I. Lower prevalence of diabetes in female former college athletes compared with non-athletes. *Diabetes* 1986; **35:** 1101–1105

4

Benefits and Risks of Exercise in Type 2 Diabetes

DINESH NAGI

Pinderfields Hospital, Wakefield, UK

INTRODUCTION

The main goals of treatment in diabetes are the relief of symptoms, prevention and treatment of acute and long-term complications and management of accompanying disorders such as hypertension and dyslipidaemia, reduction of morbidity and mortality and enhancement of quality of life. If physical activity is to be recommended for people with type 2 diabetes, it must help to fulfil some or ideally most of the therapeutic goals with minimal side-effects. Therefore, the risk–benefit ratio of physical activity must be favourable for us to recommend it as a treatment option.

A substantial proportion of patients with newly diagnosed type 2 diabetes have both micro- and macrovascular complications at the time of clinical diagnosis[1,2]. This is true, whether the disease is diagnosed in those with symptoms[1] or in asymptomatic individuals screened with repeated oral glucose tolerance tests[2]. It is, therefore, of vital importance to review the impact of physical activity on the macro- and microvascular complications of diabetes. The metabolic syndrome associated with type 2 diabetes includes central obesity, dyslipidaemia and abnormalities of fibrinolysis and coagulation, which contribute to an excess risk of coronary heart disease and

Exercise and Sport in Diabetes. Edited by Bill Burr and Dinesh Nagi.
© 1999 John Wiley & Sons Ltd.

Table 4.1. Rationale for promoting exercise in type 2 diabetes

- As an adjunct to diet for initial weight loss
- Aid in maintaining the weight loss
- Loss and redistribution of abdominal fat
- Favourable effect on glycaemic control
- Management of hypertension in diabetes
- Management of dyslipidaemia
- Improvement in general well-being

hypertension[3]. This was reviewed in detail in Chapter 3. In Western populations 25–30% of non-diabetic subjects may have features of this syndrome[4] and the proportion is higher in those with type 2 diabetes. Ferrannini *et al.* found that up to two-thirds of the non-diabetic population had one or more components of this syndrome, with only one-third of individuals being completely free[5].

Physical inactivity is related to all components of the metabolic syndrome[6,7], so it is logical to see if an increase in physical activity will have beneficial effects. It is important to know whether physical activity has benefits in addition to those due to dietary modifications, since physical activity is recommended in the initial management plan in conjunction with diet[8]. There is evidence that physical activity may improve glucose utilisation by mechanisms which differ from those of diet[9], and that the combination of diet and physical activity may be additive or synergistic[10].

Physical activity is of benefit in treating dyslipidaemia and hypertension, risk factors which contribute substantially to the excess mortality from macrovascular disease[11]. There is now an established rationale for prescribing physical activity in type 2 diabetes (Table 4.1), and the view that an increase in physical activity may benefit most patients with type 2 diabetes is becoming popular among diabetologists. This is linked to the realisation that treatment of hyperglycaemia alone does not reduce mortality from macrovascular disease.

BENEFITS OF REGULAR PHYSICAL ACTIVITY IN TYPE 2 DIABETES

Benefits of regular physical activity in type 2 diabetes have been known for years and formed the basis of ADA recommendations (Table 4.2)[12]. They are summarised in Chapter 3.

Table 4.2.   ADA recommendations for exercise in type 2 diabetes

- Lowering of blood glucose
- Increase in insulin sensitivity
- Improvement in lipid profile
- Promotion of weight gain
- Maintenance of body weight
- Reduction in dose/need for insulin or oral agents

In brief, moderate-intensity physical activity, if taken regularly and at frequent intervals, is likely to improve plasma glucose concentration in the short and long term due to beneficial effects on hepatic and peripheral insulin sensitivity. This is not surprising as the exercising muscles use 7–20 times more glucose than non-exercising muscles[13]. The long-term improvement in glycaemic control is likely to be due to the cumulative effect of repeated bouts of physical activity. It is also suggested that the improvement in fasting plasma glucose may be of larger magnitude in those on diet or oral hypoglycaemic agents than in those treated with insulin[14]. These results indicate that the best time to promote physical activity in subjects with type 2 diabetes is around the time of diagnosis, a time when motivation for behaviour change is at its highest in most subjects. There is evidence that increased physical activity in those on drug treatment for diabetes is associated with a reduction, or discontinuation, of treatment in a substantial proportion of patients[10,15]. Regular physical activity has been shown to be of benefit in promoting weight loss when used in conjunction with diet and may help to maintain weight loss in the long term[10,16].

The role of regular physical activity initiated at or around the time of diagnosis of type 2 diabetes in delaying the need for drug treatment needs to be evaluated further. Another potential role of physical activity in the clinical management of type 2 diabetes may be to limit the undesirable weight gain usually associated with initiation of sulphonylurea or insulin treatment, and this needs to be investigated.

The beneficial effects of physical activity in type 2 diabetes on dyslipidaemia and hypertension are of great importance, as successful modification of these two risk factors has been shown to reduce mortality from macrovascular disease[17], in contrast to the disappointing lack of effect of tight glycaemic control. The result of the United Kingdom Prospective Diabetes Study (UKPDS) showed that intensive blood glucose control in subjects with type 2 diabetes significantly reduced microvascular complications by 25%, while the effect on diabetes-related death and all-cause mortality was small and not significant[18]. Tight control of blood pressure to less than 144/82 mmHg was associated with highly significant reductions in diabetes-related death (32%), strokes (44%) and microvascular disease (37%)[19]. In a meta-analysis of 25 studies looking at the effects of physical activity on blood pressure, there was an average reduction of 11 and 8 mmHg, respectively, in systolic and diastolic blood pressures. This magnitude of blood pressure reduction may be particularly useful in those with mild hypertension and in early stages of the disease[20].

The effects of physical activity on lipids have been discussed in Chapter 3 and involve a reduction in triglyceride and a rise in HDL-cholesterol, both of which may be related to reduced insulin resistance[21]. There is also some reduction of LDL-cholesterol levels as well as an improvement in LDL particle density, thereby making it less atherogenic. The effects of physical activity when combined with diet are more marked than those seen with dietary modification alone.

In addition to the specific benefits on risk factors for cardiovascular disease, there are other ancillary benefits (Table 4.3).

Table 4.3. Potential benefits of regular exercise in type 2 diabetes

1. Lowers blood glucose during and after exercise
2. Increases insulin sensitivity
3. Lowers basal and post prandial insulin levels
4. Lowers glycated haemoglobin over long term
5. Lowers systolic and diastolic blood pressure
6. Quantitative and qualitative changes in circulating lipids:
   - lower triglyceride, lower LDL-cholesterol, higher HDL-cholesterol
   - beneficial effects on LDL density?
7. Improves fibrinolysis, lowers plasma fibrinogen
8. Other benefits:
   - cardiovascular conditioning
   - improves strength
   - improves sense of well-being (physical and psychological)
   - better quality of life

EFFECTS ON LONG-TERM MORTALITY

There are no long-term randomised intervention studies assessing the effect of physical activity on total and cardiovascular mortality in subjects with type 2 diabetes: such studies would have major logistical and ethical problems. In the 6-year Malmo study of an outpatient-based physical activity programme, Eriksson *et al.*[22] investigated subjects with type 2 diabetes and impaired glucose tolerance. The overall mortality in the whole cohort was 3.3% (230 of 6956 subjects), with an annual mortality figure of 0.5%. The relative risk of death in the treatment cohort with life style interventions (5 of 222 subjects) was 0.67, which was not statistically significant from the control group. However, no cases of acute myocardial infarction occurred among those who continued with the treatment protocol for a period of 6 years, which is reassuring. The cumulative mortality in subjects with IGT and type 2 diabetes who participated in the programme was 3.2%, which was significantly less than those with known diabetes (mortality 11.9%). Clearly only a limited conclusion can be drawn from this non-randomised study, but physical activity appears to be safe over a long period and may have benefits in terms of lowering mortality rates. The publication of a 12-year follow up from the same study in subjects with IGT showed that lifestyle interventions with diet and exercise achieved mortality rates similar to those in individuals with normal glucose tolerance[23].

In a meta-analysis of studies investigating the role of physical activity in relation to primary prevention of coronary artery disease in non-diabetic subjects, Berlin and Colditz[24] found that the relative risk of death comparing sedentary and non-sedentary subjects was 1.9 (95% CI 1.6–2.2). Their analysis included 27 studies of occupational and eight studies of non-occupational activity. They also suggested that the methodologically stronger studies showed a larger benefit[24]. O'Connor *et al.*[25] analysed 22 randomised studies which included physical activity as part of the rehabilitation programme following acute myocardial infarction, and found that mortality was reduced by 20%. The results were similar in studies which included physical activity alone as part of rehabilitation. These results were from studies performed in non-diabetic subjects, but there does not seem to be any good reason why the results should not be applicable to people with type 2 diabetes. They suggest that regular physical activity is likely to be of benefit in reducing mortality and prolonging life.

In non-diabetic subjects, regular physical activity is known to improve psychological well-being and overall quality of life[26]. There are no studies in subjects with type 2 diabetes, but this type of benefit is generally perceived by patients to be of equal importance to the effects on physical well-being.

RISKS OF PHYSICAL ACTIVITY

SPORTS INJURIES

Whether subjects with diabetes taking physical activity and engaging in exercise and sport are more prone to musculoskeletal injuries than non-diabetic subjects is unknown. A study with 3-year follow up showed that there was an association between sport-related ankle fractures and diabetes and obesity in middle-aged and older individuals[27] but it is unclear if the association of diabetes with ankle fracture during sport is independent of obesity. Subjects with diabetes are prone to stress fracture of the lower extremities, which may be due to the presence of neuropathy, vascular disease, and associated low bone density. Upper-extremity injuries may also be more common in subjects with diabetes and may be due to a higher prevalence of periarthritis of shoulder joints in diabetics than in those without (10.8% vs. 2.3%). These problems are frequently bilateral and are unrelated to neuropathy[28].

Musculoskeletal injuries are related to duration and intensity of physical activity. They may result from chronic, repetitive and high-impact injuries rather than actual trauma. Schneider *et al.* noticed that 12% of subjects participating in a formal exercise programme had some sort of injury, but generally these were minor[29]. It is important that these risks are discussed with the patient and appropriate steps taken to avoid them. This can be achieved by setting realistic exercise training goals and by limiting the intensity and duration of any sustained activity, particularly during exercise initiation. A period of stretching and warming-up and cooling-down periods are essential (these are highlighted in Chapter 9). Appropriate footwear and proper surroundings are also vital to minimise these risks[12].

HYPOGLYCAEMIA

The risk of hypoglycaemia applies to patients with type 2 diabetes who are treated with sulphonylureas or insulin. Hypoglycaemia may occur during or soon after physical activity, or it may be delayed for up to 24 h following a single bout of strenuous exercise, a fact not generally realised by many patients or health professionals[30]. Hypoglycaemia is not an issue in those on diet alone or taking metformin or alpha-glucosidase inhibitors. Extremely strenuous physical activity can cause transient or prolonged hyperglycaemia in type 2 diabetes, but generally only in those who are insulin deficient and have poor control of their diabetes[31].

MACROVASCULAR COMPLICATIONS

Studies have shown that a large proportion of subjects with type 2 diabetes have complications or physical disabilities which may prevent them from taking physical activity (Table 4.4)[29,32].

Samaras *et al.* found that in the non-exercising population up to 15% had diabetic foot disease, stroke or joint disease and 30% had evidence of ischaemic heart disease (IHD). They concluded that those

Table 4.4. Prevalence of complications in patients with diabetes volunteering for exercise

Complication	Prevalence (%)
Occult coronary artery disease	11
Intermittent claudication	14
Hypertension	42
Sensory neuropathy	76
Autonomic neuropathy	29
Retinopathy	16
Albuminuria:	
before exercise	8
after exercise	29

Adapted from reference 29

with IHD might not exercise due to perceived disability or risk or through discouragement by health professionals. Ironically, this group of subjects are the ones who are most likely to benefit and should be targeted for increasing physical activity[32]. In a feasibility study of exercise in patients aged 60 or over, 39 of 48 subjects with type 2 diabetes were deemed to be unfit for physical training: 14 were taking antihypertensive medication, 7 had symptoms suggestive of angina, 7 had changes on ECG but no cardiac symptoms, and 11 had locomotor dysfunction[33]. The authors concluded that most subjects in that age group could not be recommended for physical training. While 'physical training' may be an unrealistic goal in this group, none of these complications are absolute contraindications to mild or moderate-intensity aerobic physical activity, as long as the general principles of initiating physical activity are followed and individualised advice about the type of physical activity given.

Worsening of pre-existing cardiovascular disease or unmasking of previously asymptomatic CHD remains a major concern. Up to 20% of newly diagnosed subjects with type 2 diabetes may already have asymptomatic coronary artery disease[1,34]. Sudden death due to acute myocardial infarction, arrhythmias or intracerebral bleed is much dreaded but exceedingly rare, with a documented incidence of 0–2 per 1,000,000 h of exercise[35]. This risk is only slightly increased in those with pre-existing heart disease[36].

MICROVASCULAR COMPLICATIONS

In theory, strenuous physical activity could have an adverse effect on the microvascular complications of diabetes. There is no evidence that moderate-intensity physical activity has a detrimental effect on non-proliferative retinopathy and the risk in patients with proliferative retinopathy is low[37]. It seems prudent to avoid vigorous physical activity, which involves pounding, repeated jarring, weight lifting, high-impact aerobics, and activities which involve the Valsalva manoeuvre, if there is proliferative retinopathy or vitreous haemorrhage. Exercises such as walking, swimming, low-impact aerobics or stationary cycling would be appropriate in these individuals. Those with known retinopathy need to have regular retinal review depending on the severity of the retinopathy[12, 37].

Exercise is known to increase albuminuria during and in the period immediately after exercise, although the long-term implications for diabetic nephropathy are unclear[38,39]. Exercise capacity is often limited in subjects with overt nephropathy, *per se* or due to concomitant autonomic neuropathy[40]. There seems to be no good reason to restrict low- to moderate-intensity exercise in these subjects, although they should be discouraged from high-intensity strenuous physical activity. It is clearly important that in these subjects appropriate attention is paid to achieving and maintaining good glycaemic and blood pressure control. Those patients with nephropathy who are already on renal dialysis will have reduced exercise capacity, and most will have co-existing cardiac involvement. Exercise benefits should apply equally to these subjects, but physical activity programmes would need to be adjusted to the patient's complications and disabilities.

Patients should be screened for peripheral neuropathy, foot deformity or degenerative joint disease to avoid injury and adequate advice about foot care should be provided. Those who have significant neuropathy and insensitive feet are more prone to foot ulceration and fractures so that weight-bearing exercises such as step exercises and prolonged jogging or walking should be undertaken with care or avoided. Sensory involvement with Charcot arthropathy or foot ulcers is generally considered to be an absolute contraindication for weight-bearing exercises: non-weight-bearing exercises such as bicycling, swimming, rowing and arm exercises are more appropriate in these circumstances.

Patients with autonomic neuropathy may have a decreased capacity for exercise, especially high-intensity exercise, due to their inadequate cardiovascular response to exercise—such as an impaired increase in heart rate. These subjects may be more prone to episodes of extreme hypo- or hypertension following exercise, especially if exercise is vigorous[40]. Postural hypotension may be aggravated and subjects may be at risk of accumulating excess fluid loss through sweating, which may be relevant in hot climates. There are no data on the effects of exercise on long-term progression of autonomic neuropathy. Exercise in these individuals needs to be gentle and is perhaps better limited to sessions of short duration.

Despite the potentially harmful effects of exercise on micro and macrovascular complications, the benefits of exercise generally

Table 4.5.   How much exercise do we need?

- Three to five times/week, spaced at no more than 48-h intervals
- Mild- to moderate-intensity (aerobic and/or resistance training)
- 15–60 min per session, with warm-up and cool-down periods of approximately 5 min
- Brisk walking, jogging or running, swimming, cycling, tennis, badminton, skiing, dancing, etc.

---

outweigh the risks associated with it[37]. The risks can be minimised by individualisation of physical activity programmes and careful selection of patients after clinical evaluation. Advice appropriate for age, sex, ethnic and cultural background should be available to all. Those who take no regular physical activity should be told that some physical activity is better than none. Those patients wishing to increase their physical activity should be advised to start with relatively low-intensity exercise and build up gradually as physical conditioning occurs. They should be advised to limit the duration of exercise at the outset, and to report immediately any untoward symptoms. They should preferably find an activity which is enjoyable, causes no financial or physical harm and is easily accessible.

There still is no universal consensus as to the intensity and duration of physical activity which is optimal for health benefits. Recent evidence indicates that physical activity of low to moderate intensity is likely to be beneficial[41], with a combination of both aerobic and high-intensity physical activity[21]. The suggested frequency and duration of exercise is given in Table 4.5.

CONCLUSIONS

Physical activity may not be a panacea for all ailments, but it has beneficial effects on the physical and psychological well-being of patients and has the potential to improve quality of life. It has effects on glycaemic control and risk factors for cardiovascular disease that should translate into improved outcomes with reduction of mortality and prolongation of life. Evidence suggests that regular physical activity has the potential to benefit most patients with type 2 diabetes and the risk–benefit ratio of physical activity is acceptable. There continues to be a large gap between theory and practice, and sufficient emphasis is currently not being given to the multiple benefits of physical activity in subjects with type 2 diabetes and to the population in general. The advice about physical activity currently given to patients is minimal, with encouraging words such as 'exercise is good for you', or 'you should try to do more exercise'. Such platitudes are unlikely to bring about lifestyle changes. At present, little effort is being made to assess the exercise pattern of patients and to examine their potential to increase activity. With so little formal emphasis on the benefits of physical activity, it is not surprising that there is little success in modifying this aspect of patient behaviour.

Health professionals need to learn more about attitudes and barriers to exercise in patients and to educate our patients and ourselves about the health benefits of exercise. We should use our existing knowledge to promote physical activity in people with type 2 diabetes, most of whom are willing and enthusiastic but lacking proper education and help in this regard. We urgently need to assess the effectiveness of innovative approaches to increase physical activity[42]. New systems of care will require careful planning, more resources—and, above all, rigorous evaluation to review critically their benefits and cost effectiveness. We need educational programmes to provide initial patient education and prepare individuals to exercise safely on their own by choosing activities which fit into their daily lifestyle. This will allay fears and anxieties about exercise, so that they can continue exercising on their own, with less frequent contact with health professionals.

REFERENCES

1. UK Prospective Diabetes Study 6. Complications in newly diagnosed type 2 patients and their associations with different clinical and biochemical risk factors. UKPDS Group. *Diabetes Research* 1990; **13:** 1–11
2. Nagi DK, Pettitt DJ, Bennett PH, Klein R, Knowler WC. Diabetic retinopathy assessed by fundus photography in Pima Indians with impaired glucose tolerance and NIDDM. *Diabetic Med* 1997; **14:** 449–456
3. Reaven GM. Role of insulin resistance in human disease. *Diabetes* 1988; **37:** 1595–1607.

4. DeFronzo RA, Ferrannini E. Insulin Resistance: A multifaceted syndrome responsible for NIDDM, obesity, hypertension, dyslipidaemia and atherosclerotic vascular disease. *Diabetes Care* 1991; **14:** 173–194

5. Ferrannini E, Haffner, Mitchell BD, Stern MP. Hyperinsulinaemia: the key feature of a cardiovascular and metabolic syndrome. *Diabetologia* 1991; **34:** 416–422

6. Paffenbarger RS, Wing AL, Hyde RT, Jung DL. Physical activity and the incidence of hypertension in college alumni. *Am J Epidemiol* 1983; **117:** 245–257

7. Siscovick DS, Laporte RE, Newman JM. The disease specific benefits and risks of physical activity and exercise. *Public Health Rep* 1985; **100:** 180–188

8. National Institutes of Health. Consensus development conference on diet and exercise in non-insulin-dependent diabetes mellitus. *Diabetes Care* 1987; **10:** 639–644

9. Bogardus C, Ravussin E, Robbins DC, Wolfe DC, Horton ES, Sims EAH. Effects of physical training and diet therapy on carbohydrate metabolism in patients with glucose intolerance and non-insulin dependent diabetes mellitus. *Diabetes* 1984; **33:** 311–318

10. Wing RR, Epstein LH, Paternostro-Bayles M, Kriska A, Nowalk MP, Gooding W. Exercise in a behavioral weight control programme for obese patients with type II diabetes. *Diabetologia* 1988; **31:** 902–909

11. Panzram G. Mortality and survival in type 2 (non-insulin-dependent) diabetes mellitus. *Diabetologia* 1987; **30:** 123–131

12. American Diabetes Association. Clinical Practice Recommendations. Diabetes Mellitus and Exercise. *Diabetes Care* 1998; **21**(Suppl. 1): S41–S44

13. Wahren J, Felig P, Ahlborg G, Jorfeldt L. Glucose metabolism during leg exercise in man. *J Clin Invest* 1971; **50:** 2715–2725

14. Barnard J, Tiffany J, Inkeles SB. Diet and exercise in the treatment of NIDDM. *Diabetes Care* 1994; **17:** 1469–1472

15. Heath GW, Leonard BE, Wilson RH, Kendrick JS, Powell KE. Community-based exercise intervention: Zuni diabetes project. *Diabetes Care* 1987; **10:** 579–583

16. Lehmann R, Vokac A, Niedermann K, Agosti K, Spinas GA. Loss of abdominal fat and improvement of the cardiovascular risk profile by regular moderate exercise training in patients with NIDDM. *Diabetologia* 1995; **38:** 1313–1319

17. Collins R, Petro R, MacMahon S. Blood pressure, stroke, and coronary heart disease. II. Effects of short-term reductions in blood pressure: an overview of the unconfounded randomized drug trials in an epidemiological context. *Lancet* 1990; **335:** 827–838

18. UK Prospective Diabetes Study (UKPDS) Group. Intensive blood-glucose control with sulphonylurea or insulin compared with conventional

treatment and risk of complications in patients with type 2 diabetes (UKPDS 33). *Lancet* 1998; **352**: 837–853

19. UK Prospective Diabetes Study (UKPDS) Group. Tight blood pressure control and risk of macrovascular complications in type 2 diabetes (UKPDS 38). *BMJ* 1998; **317**: 703–713

20. Hagberg JM. Exercise, fitness and hypertension. In: Bouchard C (ed). *Exercise, fitness and health: a consensus of current knowledge.* Human Kinetics, Champaign, Illinois, 1990, pp. 455–456

21. Eriksson J, Taimela S, Koivisto VA. Exercise and the metabolic syndrome. *Diabetologia* 1997; **40**: 125–135

22. Eriksson KF, Lindgarde F. Prevention of type 2 (non-insulin dependent) diabetes mellitus by diet and physical exercise: the six year Malmo feasibility study. *Diabetologia* 1991; **34**: 891–898

23. Eriksson KF, Lindgarde F. No excess 12-year mortality in men with impaired glucose tolerance who participated in Malmo preventive trail with diet and exercise. *Diabetologia* 1998; **41**: 1010–1017

24. Berlin JA, Colditz GA. A meta analysis of physical activity in the prevention of coronary heart disease. *Am J Epidemiol* 1990; **132**: 612–628

25. O'Connor GT, Buring JE, Yusaf S *et al.* An overview of randomized trials of rehabilitation with exercise after myocardial infarction. *Circulation* 1989; **80**: 234–244

26. McAuley E. Physical activity and Psychological outcomes. In: Bouchard C, Shepard RG, Stephens T (eds). *Physical activity, fitness and health: international proceedings and consensus statement.* Human Kinetics, Champaign, Illinois, 1994, pp. 551–568

27. Daly PJ, Fitzgerald RH Jr, Melton LJ, Ilstrup DM. Epidemiology of ankle fractures in Rochester, Minnesota. *Acta Orthop Scand* 1987; **58**: 539–544.

28. Bridgeman JF. Periarthritis of shoulder and diabetes mellitus. *Am Rheum Dis* 1972; **31**: 69–72

29. Schneider SH, Khachadurian AK, Amorosa LF, Clemow L, Ruderman NB. Ten-year experience with an exercise-based outpatient life-style modification program in the treatment of diabetes mellitus. *Diabetes Care* 1992; **15**(Suppl. 4):1800–1810

30. MacDonald MJ. Post-exercise late-onset hypoglycaemia in insulin-dependent diabetic patients. *Diabetes Care* 1987; **10**: 584–588

31. Mitchell TH, Abraham G, Schiffrin A *et al.* Hyperglycaemia after intense exercise in IDDM subjects during continuous subcutaneous insulin infusion. *Diabetes Care* 1988; **11**: 311–317

32. Samaras K, Ashwell S, Mackintosh A-M, Campbell LV, Chisholm DJ. Exercise in NIDDM: Are we missing the point? *Diabetic Med* 1996; **13**: 780–781

33. Skarfors ET, Wegener TA, Lithell H, Selinus I. Physical training as a

treatment for type II (non-insulin dependent) diabetes in elderly men. *Diabetologia* 1987; **30:** 930–933

34. Chiariello M. Silent Myocardial ischaemia in patients with diabetes mellitus. *Circulation* 1996; **93:** 2089–2091
35. Haskell WL. Cardiovascular complications during exercise training of cardiac patients. *Circulation* 1978; **57:** 920–924
36. Debusk RF, Valdez R, Houston, N, Haskell W. Cardiovascular responses to dynamic and static efforts soon after myocardial infarction. *Circulation* 1978; **58:** 368–375
37. American Diabetes Association. Diabetes and Exercise: the risk–benefit profile. In: Devlin JT, Ruderman N (eds) *The health professionals guide to diabetes and exercise.* American Diabetes Association, Alexandria, VA, 1995, pp. 3–4
38. Mogensen CE, Vittinghus E. Urinary albumin excretion during exercise in juvenile diabetes. *Scand J Clin Lab Invest* 1975; **35:** 295–300
39. Viberti GC, Jarrett RJ, McCartney M, Keen H. Increased glomerular permeability to albumin induced by exercise in diabetic subjects. *Diabetologia* 1978; **14:** 293–300
40. Hilsted J, Galbo H, Christensen NJ. Impaired cardiovascular responses to graded exercise in diabetic autonomic neuropathy. *Diabetes* 1979; **28:** 313–319
41. Blair SN, Kohl HW, Gordon NF, Paffenbarger RS. How much physical activity is good for health. *Annu Rev Public Health* 1992; **13:** 99–126
42. Marcus BH, Simkin LR. The transtheoretical model: application to exercise behaviour. *Med Sci Sports Exerc* 1994; **26:** 1400–1404

5

Exercise in Children and Adolescents

CHRIS THOMPSON[a], ALAN CONNACHER[b], DENNIS REWT[c], and RAY NEWTON[d]

[a]Beaumont Hospital, Dublin, Republic of Ireland; [b]Perth Royal Infirmary, Perth, UK; [c]University of Edinburgh Outdoors Activities Centre, UK; [d]Ninewells Hospital, Dundee, UK

INTRODUCTION

Physical activity is an intrinsic part of everyday life for children and young adults and sporting prowess contributes greatly to the prestige accorded by young people towards their peers. Young people consistently place sportsmen and women highly in the pantheon of those they respect and wish to emulate, a relationship which is well recognised by advertising agencies who use sportsmen and women to endorse a huge range of products from designer clothes and deodorants to junk food and beverages. In contrast, lack of sporting ability or failure of young people to participate in sporting activities can lead to social isolation and loss of self-confidence. Exercise in children and young adults with insulin-dependent (type 1) diabetes mellitus can lead to profound metabolic disturbances occasionally leading to hyperglycaemia and ketosis or, more frequently, to hypoglycaemia, which can detract from the enjoyment of exercise and reduce confidence to participate, a sequence of events which can

Exercise and Sport in Diabetes. Edited by Bill Burr and Dinesh Nagi.
© 1999 John Wiley & Sons Ltd.

compound the sense of loneliness which is experienced by many young people with diabetes. The tragedy of such a scenario is that it need not be so; with a little care, education and organisation, people with type 1 diabetes can participate fully in almost any form of exercise. Moreover, as evidence accumulates that regular exercise in early life can confer protection against vascular events in later life, young patients should be actively encouraged to include physical activity in their normal daily routine, in very much the way that they are currently given dietary advice or education about blood glucose monitoring or insulin adjustment.

In this chapter we describe the pitfalls for young people with type 1 diabetes when they exercise and the strategies adopted to avoid those pitfalls. We also discuss the difficulties in encouraging young people to take regular exercise and the structures, such as camps and courses, within which the adaptations necessary for safe participation in sporting activities are provided. The greater part of our experience with sporting activities has been derived from our association with the annual camp run at Firbush Point Field Centre on the shores of Loch Tay, Scotland. Much of the practical advice included in the chapter has been developed from involvement with young people with diabetes who attend this camp. We therefore describe the structure and philosophy of this camp in order to put into context the attitudes to sport and diabetes which we espouse.

METABOLIC EFFECTS OF EXERCISE

The physiology of exercise is covered in some detail in Chapter 1. Exercise causes a dramatic increase in muscle glucose utilisation, and the need for a steady supply of substrate for energy generation. The main substrate is glucose in exercise of short duration, and this is derived from increased hepatic glycogenolysis. During sustained exercise, gluconeogenesis from lactate, alanine and glycerol assumes greater importance[1]. In the non-diabetic human, secretion of insulin from the pancreas is suppressed during exercise and there is a rise in plasma catecholamines[2], growth hormone and glucocorticoids[3]. This creates a hormonal milieu which allows mobilisation of free fatty acids from triglycerides, breakdown of hepatic glycogen stores, stimulation of gluconeogenesis and maintenance of constant plasma glucose concentrations. Blood glucose concentrations remain steady throughout prolonged exercise and for some hours after cessation of exercise.

In people with Type 1 diabetes who are exercising, the presence of their usual circulating levels of insulin inhibits hepatic glycogenolysis and gluconeogenesis, which may cause blood glucose levels to fall rapidly into the hypoglycaemic range. A reduction in insulin dosage, or extra carbohydrate consumption, or both, is required shortly before starting to exercise. On the other hand, if insulin levels are reduced too much or stopped altogether, and blood sugars are elevated, exercise can produce a dramatic increase in hyperglycaemia. This may progress to ketosis, rising blood lactate and pyruvate levels[4], and osmotic symptoms of hyperglycaemia, fatigue, muscle cramps and poor athletic performance. The potential for development of ketosis during exercise in the situation of insulin deficiency is of sufficient importance that the American Diabetes Association position statement on exercise and type 1 diabetes (Table 5.1) specifically advises against exercise in the setting of hyperglycaemia and ketosis[5].

There is evidence that exercise programmes can substantially increase insulin sensitivity in young people with diabetes with a fall in daily insulin requirements, but no overall improvement in glycaemic control, as measured by glycated haemoglobin[6]. This lack of improvement in glycaemic control may be partly related to increased carbohydrate intake in order to avoid hypoglycaemia, as many young people eat considerably more around the time of exercise.

It may also relate to the potential for exercise to cause metabolic instability, leading to both hyperglycaemia and hypoglycaemia. There is a need for careful adjustment of insulin dosage and carbohydrate intake, which can, given the erratic nature of teenage life and the random occurrence of the opportunity to partake in exercise, cause management difficulties for many young adults.

Table 5.1. American Diabetes Association guidelines for exercise in diabetes, as derived from the position statement (1990)

1. Use proper footwear, and, if appropriate, other protective equipment
2. Avoid exercise in extreme heat or cold
3. Inspect feet daily and after exercise
4. Avoid exercise during periods of poor metabolic control

ATTITUDES TO EXERCISE IN YOUNG ADULTS WITH TYPE 1 DIABETES

The role of the school is very important in encouraging participation in sport and exercise, and the attitude of the school to the child with diabetes can have a crucial effect on the child's motivation to become involved in sport. Many children play sports at home with friends but it is in school sports lessons that they are first exposed to a wide spectrum of sporting activities, and the school team is usually the first taste of competitive sport. Although it is now rare, there are still teenagers who report that they were discouraged or even banned from taking part in games lessons in school because of their diabetes. This results in a decrease in confidence and self-worth which can take years to correct. The British Diabetic Association has played a major role in improving knowledge of, and attitudes towards, diabetes in schools over recent years. Teacher training courses now cover basic medical knowledge of diabetes and fear of the condition is gradually subsiding in schools. Sporting clubs tend to be very variable in their attitudes to people with diabetes, but many of the traditional prejudices are breaking down, in part because of publicity and pressure from national diabetes associations, but largely because successful participation in sport by people with diabetes is more widely recognised.

As a child progresses towards the teenage years, exercise traditionally assumes a more central and ritualised role in daily life, though there is evidence, as we embrace the computer lifestyle, that physical exercise is declining in the teenage years. In a survey of 50 children and teenagers with type 1 diabetes, most took part in similar levels of physical exertion to non-diabetic controls, though fewer diabetic children were involved in team sports, suggesting a difficulty in mixing with other children for the purposes of exercise[7]. There is a tendency for decreased participation in sport as children get older[8]. The temptation for teenagers with diabetes to lose contact with regular exercise, because of the burden of extra preparation and precautions which they must take, is all the greater. Some young people with diabetes are sufficiently well organised and motivated to incorporate exercise into their daily routine, but most need extra motivation.

In the setting of an outpatient clinic this type of motivation is difficult to achieve. The independent practice of all the authors is to include exercise, along with diet and insulin, as part of the triad of principles which contribute to good glycaemic control and a healthy lifestyle. This entails taking a positive attitude to asking about exercise, discussing the alterations of diet and insulin which are necessary to accommodate successful participation, and encouraging continued involvement. At the time of diagnosis of diabetes, we foster the attitude that patients can continue to participate in exercise and live a normal life—often before diet and insulin injections are even mentioned. The emphasis is very much on minimising the negative aspects of the effects of diabetes on exercise by giving comprehensive advice about avoidance of hypoglycaemia, while maximising the benefits of fitness and socialising. The positive aspects of exercise can be demonstrated very clearly in the setting of the out-of-clinic activities. The examples of famous sportsmen such as Danny McGrain (Glasgow Celtic and Scotland) and Gary Mabbut (Tottenham Hotspur and England), who have achieved high levels of success in prominent sports despite the perceived disadvantage of insulin-dependent diabetes, is often helpful in demonstrating that people with diabetes can and do join in sporting activities and exercise.

Many youngsters who are insufficiently persuaded of the benefits— or safety—of exercise when advised within the slightly forbidding and hierarchical atmosphere of a hospital clinic feel much more relaxed in circumstances where their peers also have diabetes and understand what a 'hypo' is and how to treat it. Out-of-clinic events are thus perceived as a very safe context within which to start or resume exercise by young people with diabetes. The presence of medical staff helps to engender the confidence to try activities which are new or demanding, but it is the knowledge that their experience of having diabetes is shared with others which is probably a more powerful factor in the creation of a secure environment. In this respect, the availability of diabetic camps is an invaluable adjunct to traditional, hospital-based diabetes care, and in particular the foster-ing of the attitude that regular exercise is important to glycaemic control, physical fitness and general well-being. The British Diabetic Association has been funding and administering camps for young adults with diabetes since 1936 and well over 100,000 children and young adults have now attended these camps.

While the main aim of diabetic camps is simply to provide a happy and enjoyable holiday, the development of social skills[9] and the ability

to attain independent control of diabetes are also regarded as important. As nearly all camps contain some element of sport or exercise,
the knowledge and practical experience of adjusting diet and insulin
to cope with exercise are skills naturally developed as camps progress.
The experience of young people attending camps is almost invariably
positive[10] with enthusiasm for the positive attitudes encouraged at
camps being shared by the parents[11]. Some specialised camps have
included formal fitness programmes[12] or have had well defined
physical objectives[13], but most simply provide the opportunity and
environment conducive to the safe enjoyment of a wide variety of
sports and outdoor activities.

THE FIRBUSH CAMP

The Firbush Point Field Centre on Loch Tay, Scotland, is run by the
Department of Physical Education, University of Edinburgh. Since
1983 it has played host to an annual one-week diabetes outdoor
activity holiday for young adults between the ages of 16 and 22 years.
The Firbush Programme embraces the traditional aim of diabetes
camps, to provide a secure environment in which young people with
diabetes can enjoy activities, socialise with other people with diabetes
and take the educational opportunity to learn about diabetes and its
management. It also seeks to harness the benefits of association
between young adults in order to allow those who are confident
and independent to give help and encouragement to those less able to
cope with diabetic life[14]. Young people with diabetes attend from
throughout the United Kingdom; some respond to advertisements in
the British Diabetic Association journal, *Balance*, and some are referred
on from their clinic doctors or specialist nurses. The activities offered
include hillwalking, kayaking, windsurfing, sailing, mountain biking
and abseiling. Fully qualified instructors teach the techniques necessary for the activities and a medical team comprising both doctors and
specialist nurses is available for advice and troubleshooting, and for
organising educational exercises such as small group discussions and
large group seminars.

The initial aims of the Firbush Youth Diabetes Project were to train a
cadre of committed young people with diabetes who would then be in
a position to set up local diabetes groups to provide a support

network for teenagers with diabetes throughout the UK. In the early years of the camp this ethos proved to be exceptionally important in disseminating self-confidence in young people with diabetes, although this role has assumed less importance with the expansion of interest in the formation of local youth diabetes groups. The Firbush Camp has adopted more the role of a medium within which young people with diabetes can learn more about diabetes through discussion of diabetes issues with other youngsters and the adjustment of insulin and diet to meet the demands of an intensely physical week.

Many of the young people attending Firbush have never attempted the sports and activities which are available at the centre. The presence of a trained medical team providing back-up to high-quality activity instructors gives them the confidence to attempt many sports which they would never have otherwise contemplated. The atmosphere and team spirit generated in an 'all-diabetes' environment strengthens the sense of security and increases the motivation to participate. Over the last few years, the medical records from Firbush justify this confidence, as very few mishaps have been recorded. The opportunity to engage in physical activity with other people with diabetes is an important aspect of the success and popularity of Firbush, as well as similar camps such as the one run by Rowan Hillson in Eskdale[13]. In this environment there is no longer a stigma associated with insulin injections, blood testing and hypos, and there is an ability to discuss coping strategies with other youngsters with diabetes— medical staff are often regarded as knowledgeable but impractical. Young people develop the confidence to experiment with insulin and diet in order to accommodate exercise into their daily routine.

PRECAUTIONS DURING EXERCISE

Hypoglycaemia may occur during physical activity, but in addition it has recently been noted that exercise quite commonly increases insulin sensitivity for a matter of hours after activity has ceased, leading to the development of late hypoglycaemia.

HYPOGLYCAEMIA DURING EXERCISE

The fall in blood glucose concentration which accompanies exercise frequently produces hypoglycaemic symptoms, which are usually mild and easily dealt with, but which are occasionally severe, particularly if they are initially overlooked. The adrenergic surge during exercise produces symptoms which may be difficult to distinguish from hypoglycaemia—or ignored in the excitement of the moment. Frost _et al._[15] found an incidence of 85 clinical episodes of hypoglycaemia in 38 children in the first two weeks of consecutive diabetic camps. Although most episodes are mild and readily treated, severe hypoglycaemia is not uncommon, and fits have been reported[16]. The likelihood of hypoglycaemia during exercise is influenced by a variety of parameters, including the following.

Pre-exercise blood glucose concentration

Hypoglycaemia is very likely if the blood glucose concentration is < 7 mmol/l before exercise, and advice should be given to take extra rapidly absorbed carbohydrate if this is the case.

Pre-exercise plasma insulin concentration

Although plasma insulin concentrations are not measured before exercise, the greater the subcutaneous bolus injected before exercise the greater the likelihood of hypoglycaemia during, or after, the period of exercise. Frost _et al._[15], in the setting of a diabetic camp, found that hypoglycaemia occurs far more frequently when the total daily insulin dose exceeded 0.7 units/kg body weight. At the Firbush Camp, we give broad advice to reduce daily insulin dosage by 25% from day one of camp activities, though there is a wide variation in individual insulin requirements throughout the week of activities. In practice, the mean reduction in insulin is 25–30% of pre-camp dosage, and mild hypoglycaemia is still common (Table 5.2):

Our experiences at Firbush are very similar to those of the Auckland group, who run a summer camp in New Zealand for a slightly younger age group (7–12 years). This group found that hypoglycaemia was common, particularly during the first few days of camp, despite a mean reduction in daily insulin dose of 33%[17]. There was a deliberate policy not to increase carbohydrate intake in this camp. This is in direct contrast to our own policy to allow free access to carbohydrate, and to encourage an increase in carbohydrate intake to

Table 5.2. Daily insulin doses and frequency of mild hypoglycaemia at Firbush Camp 1992–1995

Day	1	2	3	4	5	6	7
Insulin dose (% of usual daily dose)	83.7	74.1	70.7	73.1	72.4	70.1	69.2
Total hypos (grade 1 and 2 only)	201	66	81	92	89	87	56

counteract the increase in energy expenditure which particularly occurs during prolonged exercise. This approach is used by other groups, and during a winter skiing camp a Finnish group reported a mean increase in calorie intake of 31%, though the daily insulin dose was reduced only by a mean of 11.8%[12].

Nature of exercise; duration and intensity

The frequency and severity of hypoglycaemia increases with the duration and intensity of exercise. Short bursts of intense activity, such as squash or aerobics, are particularly likely to cause hypoglycaemia, but in practice patients successfully anticipate the likelihood of hypoglycaemia in such sports, and prevent hypos by increasing carbohydrate intake and reducing insulin before they exercise. It is often sustained exercise which catches patients unawares: at Firbush, the activities most commonly associated with frequent and severe hypos are hillwalking, canoeing and mountain biking, which are all sports typified by intense exercise of long duration.

Extremes of temperature

Hot weather causes vasodilatation and the increased skin blood flow causes more rapid absorption of insulin from subcutaneous depots, with a consequently greater risk of hypoglycaemia. The effect of cold is even more dramatic; low temperatures are associated with shivering, which, in order to induce thermogenesis, increases metabolic rate and fuel consumption, with a resultant risk of hypoglycaemia[18]. Cold-induced hypoglycaemia is a particular feature of water sports such as canoeing and windsurfing, and extra vigilance is needed when supervising these sports, especially in adverse weather conditions.

DELAYED HYPOGLYCAEMIA

The phenomenon of hypoglycaemia with onset some hours after the cessation of exercise has been recognised for some time, but only a minority of young adults with type 1 diabetes receive formal advice about the risks of delayed hypoglycaemia, or the strategies to avoid it. In one prospective study of 300 children and teenagers attending a paediatric diabetic clinic, 15% had late post-exercise hypoglycaemia in a 2-year follow-up period, with more than half of the cases resulting in loss of consciousness or seizures, and requiring treatment with intravenous glucose or subcutaneous glucagon[19]. In a 4-year period at the Firbush Camp, 1992–1995, we witnessed six episodes of severe (grade 4) hypoglycaemia, all of which occurred in the evening, several hours after exercise had ceased. In all cases, the preceding activity had consisted of sustained exercise—hillwalking or canoeing—with several minor (grade 1 or 2) hypos during the day. The daytime hypoglycaemic reactions may be significant in this respect, as there is now evidence to suggest that frequent hypoglycaemia can reduce awareness that blood glucose concentration is falling (see below).

Nocturnal hypos after exercise are extremely disconcerting to young people with diabetes. Mild hypoglycaemia occurring during exercise is perceived as predictable, easily detected and straightforward to deal with, often without significant interference with participation. Delayed hypoglycaemia is seen as less predictable and, because it typically occurs during the night, more frightening and difficult to deal with. We regard specific advice about the existence of delayed-onset hypoglycaemia, and its prevention, as essential components of our instruction package for young people with diabetes who wish to partake in regular exercise. In particular, we stress the importance of a good snack and monitoring of blood glucose concentration before going to bed; a blood glucose concentration of <7 mmol/l is highly predictive of nocturnal hypoglycaemia and should prompt extra carbohydrate intake.

The mechanisms behind the development of delayed hypoglycaemia are complex. During even brief exercise, hepatic glucose output increases by up to fivefold in order to supply sufficient glucose to keep pace with increased utilisation by muscle[20]. This can lower liver glycogen to such an extent that it can take up to 2 days to replete glycogen stores[1]. Exercise also lowers muscle glycogen stores, which must be replaced at the expense of blood glucose. Exercise increases insulin sensitivity, and this effect can be sustained for up to 12 h or more after exertion[6]. To counteract these effects it is often necessary to reduce the dose of long-acting insulin after sustained exercise as well as increasing carbohydrate intake.

In addition to the tendency of physical activity to cause both early and late hypoglycaemia there is the problem of reduced hypoglycaemia awareness. It has recently been shown that even mild hypoglycaemia is capable of completely abolishing the sympathetic warning signs associated with severe hypoglycaemia occurring in the next 24 h. The need for careful precautions to guard against delayed hypoglycaemia cannot be over-emphasised.

FOOT CARE

It is important to stress the value of foot care in people with type 1 diabetes who exercise regularly. The American Diabetes Position statement[5] (Table 5.1) emphasises the crucial importance of proper foot care to participation in sport and exercise. Good quality footwear—whether running shoes, football boots or walking boots—which is comfortable and appropriate to the exercise in question is essential for the safe enjoyment of sports. Similarly, high-quality hosiery which can cushion the feet against repetitive trauma is recommended (e.g. Thorlo® socks). Regular foot examination should be incorporated into the routine of preparation for exercise and care after completion of exercise. Prolonged exercise may cause blistering of the feet, and supplies of blister packs should be carried.

INSULIN INJECTIONS

The influence of the site of insulin injection on exercise-induced hypoglycaemia has been the topic of some debate. It has been reported that leg exercise, in the form of cycling, can increase the rate of insulin absorption[21], and that hypoglycaemia might be avoided by injecting into non-exercising sites such as the abdomen[22], though other workers have disputed these findings[23]. We have not

Table 5.3. Timing before meals of insulin injections in patients with type 1 diabetes attending Firbush Camp

	No. (%) injecting			
	Pre-breakfast	Pre-lunch	Pre-dinner	Pre-bed
> 30 min	28(19.2)	7(7.2)	21(14.4)	25(23.1)
5–30 min	53(36.3)	11(11.3)	37(25.3)	34(31.5)
< 5 min	65(44.5)	79(81.4)	89(60.2)	49(45.4)
Total number of injections	146	97	146	108

been able to show any practical problems with any injection site in the Firbush Camp, but what is clear from our data is that only a small minority of young people with diabetes actually inject their insulin 30 minutes before meals, as is recommended (Table 5.3).

The influence of this form of 'non-compliance' with insulin on the ability to partake in exercise is speculative, though one might predict that the tendency might be for higher blood glucose values immediately after meals and lower blood glucose readings before the next meal was due. Given that a large proportion of patients with type 1 diabetes do inject immediately before meals, the emergence of insulin analogues, which are rapidly absorbed and therefore designed to be injected at the time of eating, may be a significant development (see Chapter 6).

SUMMARY

Exercise is an integral part of teenage life. In addition to the benefits of physical fitness and reduced cardiovascular risk which exercise confers on all participants, in diabetes regular exercise lowers cholesterol, increases insulin sensitivity and leads to a reduction in insulin requirements. Most importantly, exercise provides an important medium for the young person with diabetes to integrate fully into normal life in young adulthood. Although precautions are required to participate safely in sports, good education and motivation from the medical team can help the young person with diabetes to participate in almost any sporting activity and achieve standards equal to those achieved by people without diabetes.

REFERENCES

1. Wahren J, Felig P & Hagenfeldt L. Physical exercise and fuel homeostasis in diabetes mellitus. *Diabetologia* 1978; **14**: 213–222
2. Christensen NJ, Galbo H, Hansen JF, Hesse B & Richter EA. Catecholamines and exercise. *Diabetes* 1979; **28**(Suppl. 1): 58–62
3. Hartley LH, Mason JW & Hogan RP. Multiple hormonal responses to prolonged exercise in relation to physical training. *Journal of Applied Physiology* 1972; **33**: 602–606
4. Berger M *et al*. Metabolic and hormonal effects of muscular exercise in juvenile type diabetes. *Diabetologia* 1977; **18**: 355–365
5. American Diabetes Association. Diabetes and exercise; position statement. *Diabetes Care* 1990; **13**: 804–805
6. Landt KW, Campaigne BA, James FW & Sperling MA. Effects of exercise training on insulin sensitivity in adolescents with Type I diabetes. *Diabetes Care* 1985; **8**: 461–465
7. Greene SA, Thompson CJ. Exercise. In: CJH Kelnar (ed). *Childhood and adolescent diabetes*. London: Chapman & Hall; 1995, pp. 283–293
8. Boreham C, Savage JM, Primrose D, Cran G & Strain J. Coronary risk factors in school children. *Archives of Diseases in Children* 1993; **68**: 182–186
9. Thompson CJ, Greene SA & Newton RW. Camps for diabetic children and teenagers. In: CJH Kelner (ed). *Childhood and adolescent diabetes*. London: Chapman & Hall; 1995, pp. 483–492
10. McGraw RK & Travis LG. Psychological effects of a special summer camp on juvenile diabetics. *Diabetes* 1973; **22**: 217–224
11. Vyas S, Mullee MA & Kinmonth A-L. British Diabetic Association holidays—what are they worth? *Diabetic Medicine* 1987; **5**: 89–92
12. Akerblom HK, Koivukangas T & Ilkka J. Experience from a winter camp for teenage diabetics. *Acta Paediatrica Scandinavica (Supplement)* 1980; **283**: 50–52
13. Hillson RM. Diabetes outward bound mountain course, Eskdale, Cumbria. *Diabetic Medicine* 1985; **2**: 217–224
14. Newton RW, Isles T & Farquhar JW. The Firbush Project—sharing a way of life. *Diabetic Medicine* 1985; **2**: 217–224
15. Frost GF, Hodges S & Swift PGF. Dietary carbohydrate deficits and hypoglycaemia in the young diabetic on holiday. *Diabetic Medicine* 1986; **3**: 250–252
16. Swift PGF & Waldon S. Have diabetes—will travel. *Practical Diabetes* 1990; **7**: 101–104

17. Braatveldt GD, Midenhall L, Patten C & Harris G. Insulin requirements and metabolic control in children with diabetes mellitus attending a summer camp. *Diabetic Medicine* 1997; **14:** 258–261
18. Gale E, Bennet T, Green GH & MacDonald I. Hypoglycaemia, hypothermia and shivering in man. *Diabetes Care* 1987; **10:** 584–588
19. MacDonald MJ. Post-exercise late-onset hypoglycaemia in insulin-dependent diabetic patients. *Diabetes Care* 1987; **10:** 584–588
20. Wahren J, Felig P, Ahlborg G & Jorfeldt L. Glucose metabolism during leg exercise in man. *Journal of Clinical Invesigation* 1971; **50:** 2712–2725
21. Dandona P, Hooke D & Bell J. Exercise and insulin absorption from subcutaneous tissue. *British Medical Journal* 1978; **1:** 479–481
22. Koivisto VA & Felig P. Effects of leg exercise on insulin absorption in diabetic patients. *New England Journal of Medicine* 1978; **298:** 79–83
23. Kemmer FW, Berchtold P, Berger M *et al.* Exercise induced fall in blood glucose concentration is unrelated to alteration of insulin metabolism. *Diabetes* 1979; **28:** 1131–1137

6

The Role of Short-Acting Insulin Analogues in Sport

VEIKKO KOIVISTO

Lilly Research Laboratories, Hamburg, Germany

INTRODUCTION

Physical exercise has traditionally been recommended as an important component of diabetic treatment. These recommendations were based on the blood-glucose-lowering effect of exercise. In recent years, data have accumulated suggesting a number of other beneficial effects of exercise in diabetic patients: patients involved in regular training have fewer complications and live longer than physically inactive patients[1]. Although these data are from cross-sectional studies and do not necessarily prove causality, they indicate that involvement in exercise is related to a better prognosis. Epidemiological surveys indicate that people with diabetes do not have less wish to do physical exercise than non-diabetics, but more than 50% of diabetic patients are not meeting physical activity goals. They need to be encouraged to exercise according to their capabilities and wishes, taking note of any physical limitations[2]. Physical activity may also have a number of benefits for diabetic children and adolescents, as discussed in Chapter 5. An important factor controlling the glycaemic response to exercise in insulin-treated diabetic patients is the insulin concentration at the time of exercise[3]. A new short-acting insulin

Exercise and Sport in Diabetes. Edited by Bill Burr and Dinesh Nagi.
© 1999 John Wiley & Sons Ltd.

analogue (insulin lispro or Humalog) has been recently introduced. As the pharmacokinetic characteristics of this analogue differ from those of human insulin, the glycaemic response to exercise is also different with the use of Humalog than it is with human soluble insulin. This chapter will focus on the new short-acting insulin analogue and its use in the treatment of exercising diabetic patients.

BLOOD GLUCOSE RESPONSE TO EXERCISE

Exercise-induced hypoglycaemia is a well known complication of insulin therapy[3,4]. The metabolic and hormonal response to exercise in patients with type 1 diabetes is determined by several factors. These include the intensity and duration of exercise, the patient's level of metabolic control, the type and dose of insulin injected before the exercise, the site of insulin injection, and the timing of the previous insulin injection and meal relative to the exercise. Depending on the interplay of all these factors, blood glucose concentrations can decline, increase or remain unchanged during exercise in insulin-treated diabetic patients (Table 6.1).

Table 6.1. Factors determining glycaemic response to acute exercise in type 1 diabetic patients

Blood glucose decreases if:
- Hyperinsulinaemia exists during exercise
- Exercise is prolonged (> 30–60 min) or intensive
- More than 3 h have elapsed since the preceding meal
- No extra snacks are taken before or during the exercise

Blood glucose remains unchanged if:
- Exercise is short
- Plasma insulin concentration is normal
- Appropriate snacks are taken before and during exercise

Blood glucose increases if:
- Hypoinsulinaemia exists during exercise
- Exercise is strenuous
- Excessive carbohydrate is taken before or during exercise

HYPERINSULINAEMIA DURING EXERCISE

The underlying reason for the excessive fall in blood glucose during exercise is hyperinsulinaemia[3]. In healthy humans, pancreatic insulin secretion falls during exercise. This cannot occur in patients treated with insulin injections and the patient often has elevated serum insulin concentrations. Hyperinsulinaemia may occur for several reasons. Firstly, short-acting insulin injected a few hours previously may exert its peak action during exercise. This effect is exaggerated if the previously injected limb is exercised, as insulin absorption is accelerated by exercise[5]. Moreover, the use of long-acting insulin generally produces higher peripheral insulin levels than normal. If exercise is performed in a warm environment and insulin has been injected in the exercising leg, both high external temperature and increased blood flow in the leg can stimulate insulin absorption[6]. Consequently, both the rise in plasma insulin and the fall in blood glucose during exercise are increased compared with exercise performed in cool temperature[6]. If serum insulin concentration is higher than normal during exercise, hyperinsulinaemia stimulates glucose uptake by the exercising muscle. In addition, hyperinsulinaemia prevents an appropriate rise in hepatic glucose production to meet the needs of exercising muscles. As a consequence, glucose utilization exceeds glucose production and hypoglycaemia ensues (Figure 6.1). Hyperinsulinaemia also prevents the normal increase in lipid mobilization during exercise, leading to reduced availability of free fatty acids as a fuel.

INSULIN LISPRO (HUMALOG)

A new short-acting insulin analogue, insulin lispro (Humalog) has been synthesized by switching the order of lysine and proline at positions B28 and B29 in the insulin B chain. As a result the insulin analogue has much less tendency for self-association than human insulin. When insulin is in the vial or cartridge, it is in a polymeric form to maintain stability. After subcutaneous injection the polymer dissociates before insulin is absorbed through the capillary wall into circulation. Humalog polymers dissociate much faster, and the insulin is absorbed much quicker, than human soluble insulin. The peak

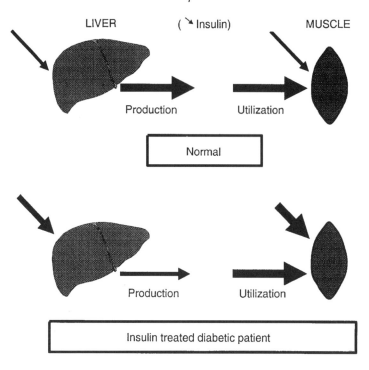

Figure 6.1. The importance of insulin in the regulation of hepatic glucose production and glucose utilization in muscle. Hyperinsulinaemia further enhances the exercise-stimulated glucose uptake by the muscle and prevents an appropriate rise in hepatic glucose production. As a consequence hypoglycaemia ensues. Modified from reference 3 by permission

insulin concentration after Humalog injection occurs faster, is higher and is of shorter duration than that following human soluble insulin injection (Figure 6.2)[7-9].

The peak hypoglycaemic activity occurs approximately 1 h after insulin lispro injection and has virtually disappeared by 4 h after the injection, whereas the hypoglycaemic activity of human insulin lasts 6–8 h after subcutaneous injection (Figure 6.3).

This difference in pharmacokinetics affects the blood glucose response to exercise taken within a few hours of the injection of short-acting insulin. Humalog was approved for clinical use in 1996 by the European Medicines Evaluation Agency (EMEA) for European countries, and by the Food and Drug Administration (FDA) for clinical use in the USA. The clinical trials have demonstrated that

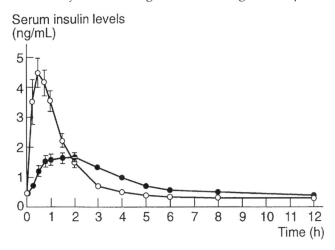

Figure 6.2. Serum insulin concentrations after subcutaneous injection of Humalog (O) or human soluble insulin (●). There are three differences in the pharmacokinetics between the two insulins: a faster absorption, a higher peak and a faster disappearance from the circulation after Humalog than after human soluble insulin. These differences are due to a lesser tendency for self-association of Humalog molecules at the injection site. Modified from reference 7, by permission

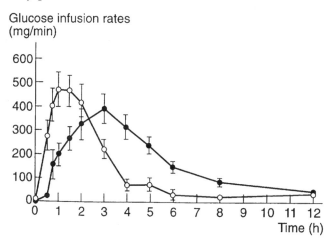

Figure 6.3. The pharmacodynamic activity profile of Humalog (O) and human soluble insulin (●) after a subcutaneous injection. These differences reflect the differences in the pharmacokinetics of the two insulins: a faster start of activity, a higher peak activity and a faster disappearance of the activity with the analogue. Thus the activity profile of Humalog is more closely related to mealtimes and the early post-prandial period

compared with human soluble insulin Humalog has several benefits: it decreases the postprandial rise in blood glucose[10], reduces both moderate[11] and severe hypoglycaemia[12], improves long-term control (HbA1c)[13] and pleases patients[14] (Table 6.2). Because the use of Humalog is steadily increasing in the therapy of insulin treated diabetic patients it is appropriate to consider the use of short-acting insulin analogue in exercising patients.

INSULIN LISPRO DURING EXERCISE

We have recently performed a study comparing the blood glucose response to exercise in type 1 diabetic patients using either human soluble insulin or insulin lispro as pre-meal therapy[15]. Ten type 1 diabetic patients participated in the study. All the patients took four injections per day as their usual daily therapy: soluble human insulin before breakfast, lunch and dinner, and intermediate-acting basal insulin either at bedtime alone or at bedtime and before breakfast. Each patient performed the exercise study four times: at times of both peak and low insulin action while treated with either human soluble insulin (Humulin Regular) or insulin lispro. Each study was started after an overnight fast at 7.30 a.m. After baseline venous samples were

Table 6.2. Comparison of the characteristics of the short-acting insulin analogue (insulin lispro or Humalog) with those of human soluble insulin

---

- Less tendency for self-association at the injection site compared with human soluble insulin. Consequently, it is absorbed faster, has a higher peak and disappears faster from the circulation than soluble human insulin
- Decreases the postprandial rise in blood glucose
- Can be injected within 15 min of the meal
- Reduces both moderate and severe hypoglycaemia
- Offers potential to improve long-term control
- Provides better treatment satisfaction
- The fall in blood glucose during exercise depends on the time interval between the Humalog injection and exercise
- If exercise is performed within 2 h of the Humalog injection, reduce the dose by 20–30%

---

taken, patients injected their usual morning insulin, which in each study was the same: 6.3($\pm$0.8) U of either Humulin Regular or the insulin analogue. The three patients who received intermediate-acting insulin in the morning injected their usual dose (11.7($\pm$3.0) U) of Humulin NPH insulin from the same syringe. All the injections were given subcutaneously in the abdomen. A standard breakfast (550 kcal, 40 g carbohydrate) was eaten 30 min after the injection of Humulin Regular insulin and 5 min after the analogue injection; 120 min later, a snack (30 g carbohydrate) was taken. Breakfast time is taken as time 0. A 40-min cycle ergometer exercise (load $\sim$80 W, heart rate $\sim$130 beats/min, peak blood lactate 2.3 mmol/l, similar in all studies) was performed either 40 min (early exercise) or 180 min (late exercise) after breakfast. The first two studies were done when patients were using Humulin Regular, and the last two when using insulin analogue. The interval between early and late exercise studies with the same insulin preparation was one week.

Insulin lispro was able to prevent totally a post-breakfast rise in plasma glucose, which occurred with human soluble insulin (Figure 6.5).

When exercise was performed 40 min after breakfast, the exercise-induced fall in plasma glucose was 2.2-fold greater ($P < 0.01$), whereas during late exercise the fall in plasma glucose was 46% less ($P < 0.05$) after the analogue than after Humulin Regular (Figure 6.6).

Fasting serum insulin concentrations were similar in all studies (Figure 6.4). After insulin lispro injection, serum insulin concentrations peaked earlier, to a level which was 56% higher ($P < 0.05$), and which decreased faster than after human insulin (Figure 6.4).

Thus, when the analogue was used hyperinsulinaemia was greater during early exercise and tended to be lower during late exercise. The fall in plasma glucose during early exercise correlated with serum human insulin or insulin lispro concentration, as determined in the beginning of the exercise (Figure 6.7).

The early exercise was performed during peak insulin concentrations. Owing to higher insulin concentrations, insulin lispro caused a more than two-fold greater fall in blood glucose compared with human soluble insulin treatment. The importance of insulin for the hypoglycaemic response is supported by the close correlation between serum insulin concentration at the beginning of exercise

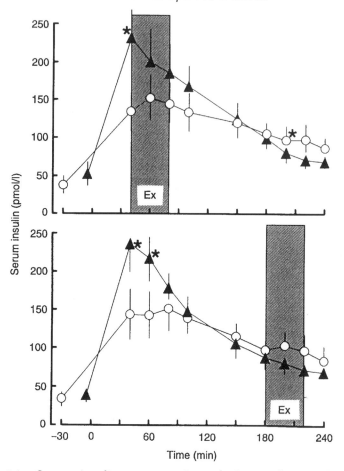

Figure 6.4. Serum insulin concentrations during early exercise (EX) are higher after the injection of insulin lispro (▲) than after soluble human insulin (○), whereas the situation is the opposite during late exercise. Soluble insulin was injected 30 min and lispro 5 min after breakfast, and the exercise was started 40 min (early) or 180 min (late) after breakfast. *$P < 0.05$. From reference 15, by permission

and the subsequent fall in blood glucose. During late exercise, serum insulin concentrations were slightly lower after the analogue than after human soluble insulin. Consequently, the hypoglycaemic effect of exercise was smaller in the patients treated with the analogue than those using human soluble insulin.

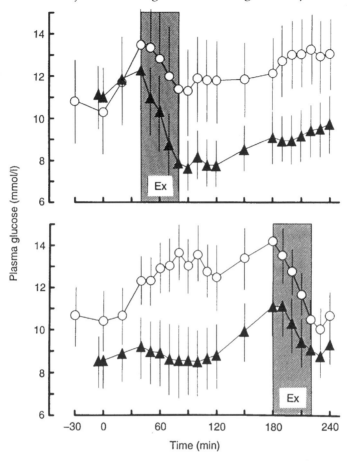

Figure 6.5. The fall in plasma glucose is greater during early exercise after insulin lispro (▲) injection, when the insulin level is high (see Figure 6.4), but less during late exercise after insulin lispro injection, when the serum insulin concentration is lower compared to soluble human insulin (○) From reference 15, by permission

Thus, compared with soluble human insulin, the much faster absorption of the insulin analogue can either augment or reduce the fall in plasma glucose during exercise, depending on the interval between insulin injection and the time of exercise. These pharmacokinetic characteristics are important to know, when insulin lispro or other short-acting insulin analogues are used.

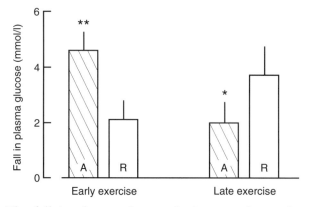

Figure 6.6. The fall in plasma glucose during exercise performed either 45 min (early exercise) or 180 min (late exercise) after breakfast. Insulin lispro (A) was injected 5 min and human soluble insulin (R) 30 min before the breakfast. *$P < 0.05$, **$P < 0.01$. From reference 15, by permission

SUMMARY

A new short-acting insulin analogue, insulin lispro or Humalog, where proline and lysine are reversed in the B-chain positions 28 and 29, has a lesser tendency for self-association than human soluble insulin. As a consequence, this analogue is absorbed faster, gives a higher peak insulin concentration and more rapid fall of serum insulin than soluble human insulin. The more precise time action profile during and after meals prevents post-prandial hyperglycaemia better than soluble insulin. The exercise-induced change in plasma glucose depends on the prevailing insulin concentration. In comparison with Humulin soluble insulin, the fall in blood glucose is greater if the exercise is performed soon (45 min), but smaller if the exercise occurs late after the insulin injection and the meal. If the patient is using Humalog and exercise is performed soon after the meal, the pre-meal insulin dose should be reduced. If exercise is taken later after the meal (which is often the case), the fall in plasma glucose is less in the patients using Humalog than in those using human soluble insulin. In order to get the maximal benefits from the new short-acting insulin analogue, it is important for health care professionals and patients to learn the pharmacokinetic characteristics of the new analogue.

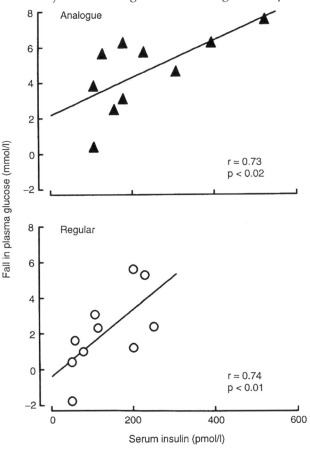

Figure 6.7. Correlation between insulin lispro concentration (upper panel) and human insulin concentration (lower panel) in early exercise and the fall in plasma glucose during early exercise. From reference 15, by permission

REFERENCES

1. Moy CS, Songer TJ, LaPorte R *et al*. Insulin-dependent diabetes mellitus, physical activity, and death. *Am J Epidemiol* 1993; **137:** 74–81
2. Ford ES, Herman WH. Leisure-time physical activity patterns in the U.S. Diabetic population. Findings from the 1990 National Health Interview Survey—Health Promotion and Disease Prevention Supplement. *Diabetes Care* 1995; **18:** 27–33

3. Vranic M, Berger M. Exercise and diabetes mellitus. *Diabetes* 1979; **28**: 147–63

4. Lawrence RD. The effect of exercise on insulin action in diabetes. *Br Med J* 1926; **1**: 648–650

5. Koivisto VA, Felig P. Effects of leg exercise on insulin absorption in diabetic patients. *N Engl J Med* 1978; **298**: 79–83

6. Rönnemaa T, Koivisto VA. Combined effect of exercise and ambient temperature on insulin absorption and postprandial glycemia in type 1 diabetes. *Diabetes Care* 1988; **11**: 769–773

7. Howey DC, Bowsher RR, Brunelle RL, Woodworth JR. [Lys(B28), Pro(B29)]-human insulin. A rapidly absorbed analog of human insulin. *Diabetes* 1997; **43**: 396–402

8. Holleman F, Hoekstra JBL. Insulin lispro. *N Engl J Med* 1997; **337**: 176–183

9. Wilde MI, McTavish D. Insulin lispro. A review of its pharmacological properties and therapeutic use in the management of diabetes mellitus. *Drugs* 1997; **54**: 597–614

10. Anderson JH Jr, Brunelle RL, Koivisto VA, Trautmann ME, Vignati L, DiMarchi R. Improved mealtime treatment of diabetes mellitus using an insulin analogue. *Clin Ther* 1997; **19**: 62–72

11. Anderson JH, Brunelle RL, Koivisto VA, Pfützer A, Trautmann M, Vignati R, DiMarchi R and the Multicenter Insulin Lispro Study Group. Reduction of postprandial hyperglycemia and frequency of hypoglycemia in IDDM patients on insulin-analog treatment. *Diabetes* 1997; **46**: 265–270

12. Brunelle RL, Llewelyn J, Anderson JH Jr, Gale EAM, Koivisto VA. Meta-analysis of the effect of insulin lispro on severe hypoglycaemia in patients with type 1 diabetes. *Diabetes Care* 1998; **21**: 1726–1731

13. Ebeling P, Jansson PA, Smith U, Lalli C, Bolli GB, Koivisto VA. Strategies toward improved control during insulin lispro therapy in IDDM. Importance of basal insulin. *Diabetes Care* 1997; **20**: 1287–1289

14. Kotsanos JG, Vignati L, Huster W *et al.* Health-related quality-of-life results from multinational clinical trials of insulin lispro. *Diabetes Care* 1997; **20**: 948–958

15. Tuominen JA, Karonen S-L, Melamies L, Bolli G, Koivisto VA. Exercise-induced hypoglycemia in IDDM patients treated with a short-acting insulin analogue. *Diabetologia* 1995; **38**: 106–111

7

Specific Sports

CHRIS THOMPSON[a] and BILL BURR[b]

[a]Beaumont Hospital, Dublin, Republic of Ireland; [b]Pinderfields Hospital, Wakefield, UK

GENERAL PRINCIPLES

The basic principles for making insulin dose reductions, and for taking extra carbohydrate when exercising, were outlined in Chapter 2. When trying to calculate the energy expenditure in different sports, a number of different variables have to be taken into account:

1. Type of activity
2. Duration
3. Physique of individual—the greater the body weight, the greater the energy expenditure during exercise
4. Experience of individual—beginners in many sports, for instance skiing, expend much more energy than those who are experienced
5. Weather conditions—more energy is expended in cold or windy conditions
6. Level of competition—a great deal more effort is likely to be put into a cup-final than a training match

To compare the intensity of different sporting activities, a rating system has been devised which compares the intensity of a given activity with the resting metabolic rate. This is taken to be that of an adult sitting quietly, and is defined as one MET (which for an average

Exercise and Sport in Diabetes. Edited by Bill Burr and Dinesh Nagi.
© 1999 John Wiley & Sons Ltd.

Table 7.1. Comparative energy expenditure for different sporting activities

Activity	METS	energy expenditure	
		(kcal/min)	(kcal/hour)
Walking (3 mph) Cycling (6 mph) Golf (pulling trolley)	3.5–4.0	4–5	240–300
Tennis, doubles Golf (carrying clubs) Volleyball Walking (4 mph) Mowing lawn, hand mower	4.0–6.0	5–6	300–360
Roller skating Cycling (12 mph) Jogging (5 mph) Tennis, singles Skiing (downhill, vigorous) Aerobics (high impact)	7.0–8.0	7–8	420–480
Cycling, racing Running (6–7 mph) Swimming (crawl, fast) Soccer Rugby	9.0–11.0	10–12	600–660
Squash Rock Climbing Canoeing, vigorous Skindiving Running (8–9 mph)	12.0–14.0	12 or more	720 or more

Adapted from Ainsworth *et al.*[1], by permission

adult is approximately 3.5 ml oxygen/kg body weight/min, or 1 kcal/kg body weight/h[1]. The MET value for various activities assesses their intensity in relation to the resting value of one MET (Table 7.1). For interest, this table also includes the calorie expenditure per minute and hour while performing different tasks.

By combining the information contained in Table 7.1 with the precise details of insulin dose adjustments given in Chapter 2, it should be possible to calculate the alterations of diet and insulin required for most sporting activities.

More detailed advice for selected activities now follows.

CANOEING

Canoeing, or kayaking, can, depending upon the duration of paddling, exert considerable demands upon carbohydrate stores. Long-distance paddling, particularly on the open sea, can rapidly exhaust available glucose, whereas the short-lived intensity of white-water canoeing can cause rapid falls in blood glucose concentrations. Canoeing ranks second only to hillwalking in frequency of causing hypoglycaemia. The likelihood of hypoglycaemia is increased if the canoeist becomes cold and wet, which is usually the case in this sport, so precautions need to be taken to ensure safe participation.

As with all sports, it is important to reduce insulin and take extra carbohydrate before starting canoeing. Whilst canoeing, the best way to store carbohydrate for regular 'top-ups' is either to secrete dextrose tablets up the sleeve of a wetsuit or to store chocolate bars in a waterproof bag in the zip pocket of a waterproof overjacket. Because canoeing is particularly prone to causing hypoglycaemia, and because hypoglycaemia can suddenly lead to capsizing the canoe, it is advisable to canoe with a 'buddy' who can recognise and deal with hypoglycaemia and who can effect emergency rescue techniques.

Some canoeists suggest that hypoglycaemia is more frequent if insulin is injected into the arms on the morning of the paddle, although the practical importance of this is open to debate (see Chapter 2). Significant hypoglycaemia on the evening after a paddle is a frequent problem, and adequate carbohydrate should be ingested with the evening meal and before bed.

GOLF

Golf is often considered, even by players themselves, to be a sport which is not associated with much energy expenditure. Among the sports which we will discuss, it is the one most likely to be enjoyed by people with type 2 diabetes, because of both the nature of the sport and the age group which most commonly plays golf. People with type

2 diabetes who have played golf will, however, be able to confirm that it involves considerable energy expenditure, so that someone with well controlled type 2 diabetes who embarks on a round of golf without taking any precautions will be very likely to experience symptoms of hypoglycaemia. This really should not cause any surprise because, although golf does not normally involve intense effort, the moderate effort is sustained continuously for 4 h or more. Add to this the fact that it is not customary to consume any food during a round of golf, and that there may be additional energy expenditure when carrying one's own clubs or when playing on a hilly course, and the possibilities for hypoglycaemia become very clear. In fact, players with type 2 diabetes usually find that they need to take additional carbohydrate, such as a chocolate bar, after the first nine holes, when playing a full round. Players who have insulin-treated diabetes should follow the guidelines for low-to-moderate-intensity exercise outlined in Chapter 2, with suitable adjustments on the basis of playing speed, nature of the course (hilly or not), weather conditions (wind, temperature), and whether or not carrying clubs. Table 7.1 may help in assessing the intensity of exertion, but for a 4-h round it may be necessary to reduce prandial insulin by 20–30%, and basal insulin by up to 40–50%, as well as taking extra carbohydrate after nine holes (see Chapter 2).

HILLWALKING

Hillwalking presents a considerable challenge to the individual with type 1 diabetes. The nature of the exercise, which is both prolonged and strenuous, requires not only a reasonable level of physical fitness but also considerable reduction in insulin dose and marked increases in carbohydrate intake to avoid hypoglycaemia. Hillwalking is more likely to cause hypoglycaemia than any other form of outdoor pursuit, and is particularly likely to cause delayed hypoglycaemia in the evening or the night after a hill climb has been completed. In addition, hillwalking carries the risk of foot blisters, which necessitates appropriate footwear and good foot care.

The following are guidelines for people with insulin-treated diabetes who wish to participate in hillwalking. They are not intended to be comprehensive, and they should be regarded as additional to general advice about walking and climbing in mountainous country.

1. Good equipment is essential. Appropriate walking boots which fit comfortably minimise the risk of ankle injuries and blistering. In our experience, blisters are best avoided when a pair of thin socks is worn under the thick walking socks traditionally worn on the hills. Warm, waterproof overclothes should be carried, even in good weather, as conditions can change rapidly on the hills. The combination of exercise and cold-induced shivering quickly lowers blood glucose into the hypoglycaemic range and it is important not to become cold.

2. It is not recommended that people with diabetes attempt significant climbs alone, and they ideally should climb or walk with someone who has some experience of recognising and treating hypoglycaemia. A note of the intended route and estimated time of return should be left with someone reliable before departure.

3. Insulin dose. The change in insulin dose required to avoid hypoglycaemia varies widely between individuals and depends to some extent on the preceding glycaemic control; patients who are not well controlled may develop marked hyperglycaemia and ketosis if insulin dosages are reduced by too much. Advice must be given on an individual basis, but the experience of the Firbush Project (Chapter 5) shows that insulin dose needs to be reduced by 25–30% on average. This applies equally to the dose of insulin on the evening after completing a climb, in order to avoid delayed hypoglycaemia, particularly nocturnal hypoglycaemia. Nocturnal hypoglycaemia, occurring without warning, is more likely to occur if there have been hypoglycaemic attacks during the day. The recent introduction of insulin analogues which can be injected immediately before eating without detriment to post-prandial blood glucose control is proving very useful in the setting of hillwalking. Climbers on conventional soluble insulin face the dilemma of injecting as recommended, half an hour before eating and risking hypoglycaemia while walking or climbing to the meal site, or injecting just before eating, in conflict with medical advice. In practice, most climbers opt for safety with the latter option, but the availability of insulin analogues eradicates this dilemma and many patients with insulin-treated diabetes who are regular walk-

ers or climbers have elected to switch to insulin analogues (see Chapter 6).

4. Carbohydrate intake. Hillwalking requires considerable energy expenditure, and carbohydrate intake should be increased to provide the necessary fuel and to avoid hypoglycaemia. It is crucially important to have a high-carbohydrate breakfast. The traditional eggs, bacon and sausage breakfast does not provide sufficient carbohydrate, and breakfast should comprise mainly cereal and toast, with baked beans or porridge to give a warm start in cold weather. Calorific intake needs to be maintained while walking and we find that a mixture of bananas, raisins, energy bars and chocolate provides a palatable and easily portable variety. Formal meals, such as lunch, should be bigger than usual, and it is important to stress the need for a decent evening meal and a snack before bed to prevent nocturnal hypoglycaemia. Fluid—water is preferable, though isotonic drinks are popular—should also be carried in quantities adequate for the duration of the climb and prevailing climate.

5. Blood glucose monitoring is an integral part of playing sport for people with diabetes, but it is essential that blood glucose should be checked regularly during hillwalking, in view of the high risk of hypoglycaemia. Blood glucose should always be checked before ascending a hill and urinary ketones measured if the blood glucose is greater than 17 mmol/l. Hill climbing should not be attempted while insulin deficient, as ketones are rapidly generated leading to muscle cramps, polyuria and exhaustion. If small amounts of ketones are present a small bolus of soluble insulin should be taken, but if anything more than trace ketonuria is detected consideration should be given to abandoning the climb.

ROWING

Competition rowing is among the most strenuous activities listed in Table 7.1. The precautions required for rowers with diabetes are generally similar to the advice given for canoeing. Rowing is generally an 'explosive' effort, usually sustained for about 6 min and not maintained for longer than 20–30 min at full intensity. While it is somewhat less likely than canoeing to involve complete immersion, there is still a requirement to have a safe, dry, accessible stowage place for glucose tablets or drinks for use in emergency.

For competitions, the main need is to ensure that diabetes is under reasonable control (blood glucose < 14 mmol/l and no ketones), and that a high-carbohydrate meal is taken about 2 h before the event, with a moderate reduction of short-acting insulin before the race. Training sessions are likely to be of longer duration, and may require greater reductions in insulin dose both before and after the session.

CASE HISTORY: STEVE REDGRAVE

Olympic oarsman Steve Redgrave was holder of the gold medal for coxless pairs (won at Atlanta, 1996), when he suddenly developed diabetes in October 1997, at the age of 36[2]. Although the onset was quite dramatic, and blood glucose was in excess of 20 mmol/l, he had a family history of type 2 diabetes, and eventually turned out to have developed this type himself. The condition could be controlled by sulphonylurea treatment, but this produces a constant stimulus to insulin secretion, which did not suit the variable demand for insulin imposed by Steve's training regime. He prefers to control his diabetes with five or six daily injections of the short-acting insulin analogue lispro (Humalog, see Chapter 6), because the typical twice-daily injection routine used for people with type 2 diabetes was also too inflexible. Steve initially considered abandoning his plans to continue competing until the Olympics in 2000, but eventually decided that he was not going to let diabetes make this decision for him.

He finds that Humalog gives him flexibility together with precise control of blood glucose. 'Ideally, I eat what I want, the insulin acts and is out of my system before the next training session. But when you are training all day, it can be hard to find a time to inject that won't affect the next training session, so I tend to balance it with the last injection of the day, snacking before bed. The first session's the hardest, so if I have got the glucose level right overnight, I don't need any insulin in the morning, because the training brings the levels down anyway. Before the second session I have a snack and do a test; as it tends to be less physical, and glucose levels fall less, I take a little insulin.'

He carries glucose tablets or drinks on the water, but has not had problems while training. 'Long distance races will be the biggest challenge, and on those days I reckon I will have to allow a higher blood glucose level.' Knowledge that other people have overcome the problems associated with diabetes and elite sport has been helpful. 'There's a guy with diabetes in the German Eight who came fourth at the last world championships, which helped to prove that you can still compete at high levels.'

As an athlete, Steve was already aware of his dietary needs, and found diabetes perhaps less of an imposition than other people. 'It's definitely an advantage being a sportsman. You have to be very disciplined about your whole lifestyle. Diabetes is just another part of the equation. It's not difficult—it's a pain in the neck, but that's all really.'

SOCCER AND RUGBY

Soccer and rugby rarely present problems to people with insulin-treated diabetes. If insulin is reduced—usually by 25–30%—before the game, and extra carbohydrate is taken before playing, at half-time, and at the end of the game, hypoglycaemia is not common. Most players take carbohydrate, usually in the form of dextrose tablets or isotonic drinks, to be left on the touchline in case of hypoglycaemia during a game. Delayed hypoglycaemia tends to be more of a problem, particularly after hard, prolonged evening training sessions; training is often more intense than the match itself, where there may be periods of rest. As evening training often terminates with alcoholic beverages, the combination of hard exercise, alcohol and delayed or missed meals can lead to significant hypoglycaemia, particularly at night. Hypoglycaemia can be avoided by ensuring that a meal rich in complex carbohydrate—preferably pasta-based—is taken after training has finished and by moderating alcohol intake.

TENNIS

Although tennis is characterised by periods of high-intensity exercise, the metabolic demands of even high-level competition are those of moderate-intensity, sustained exercise[3]. Table 7.1 highlights the difference between singles and doubles, the former having an energy expenditure equivalent to 8 METS, and the latter being equivalent to 6 METS.

Tennis rarely causes major metabolic disturbances in people with insulin-treated diabetes, although, as with other sports, due consideration has to be given to variables such as time in relation to last meal and insulin injection, type and dosage of insulin, amount and type of food taken, duration and intensity of match, and time of day.

Hypoglycaemia occurring during, or up to 4–6 h after, the match is the most common problem, and is relatively easily avoided by a pre-match check of blood glucose and by taking readily absorbed carbohydrate before, during and after the match. It is also advisable to make modest reductions in the dose of insulin, especially for prolonged matches, following the principles outlined in Chapter 2.

RESTRICTIONS IMPOSED BY SPORTS' GOVERNING BODIES

In general, our philosophy is to encourage participation in all forms of sport and exercise, but it should be acknowledged that there are restrictions placed by sports' governing bodies on participation by people treated with insulin.

PARTICIPATION BANNED

There are a small number of sports in which people with diabetes are not allowed to participate, and these are summarised in Table 7.2.

Table 7.2. Restrictions imposed by sports' governing bodies on participation for people with insulin-treated diabetes

Some restrictions	Total ban on participation
Ballooning	Bobsleigh
Gliding	Boxing
Motorcycle racing	Flying
Parachuting	Horse Racing*
Power boat racing	Motor car racing
Rowing	Paragliding
Underwater swimming	

*Under review

Boxing

The Amateur Boxing Association does not allow people with diabetes, whether on insulin, oral hypoglycaemic agents or diet alone, to box. All applicants must have a medical before boxing and if diabetes is diagnosed the applicant is automatically disqualified. The obvious concern is the ability of an individual to defend himself if he becomes hypoglycaemic, but there is also considerable anxiety about the effects that 'wasting'—losing weight before a bout in order to fight in a certain weight bracket—would have on control of diabetes. The Amateur Boxing Association does run a beginners' achievement course which involves no physical contact, but is designed to promote exercise and develop moral and ethical behaviour, and this is open to people with diabetes.

Judo

There are no restrictions imposed by the British Judo Association upon people with diabetes. Application forms are used by all Martial Arts clubs and if applicants declare that they have a 'chronic condition' such as diabetes, a medical certificate, mainly for insurance purposes, is required from a qualified medical practitioner which 'clears' the applicant to participate.

Flying

People with insulin-treated diabetes will not be issued with a flying licence, though people on oral hypoglycaemics can hold a private licence but must fly with a co-pilot.

Parachuting

Parachute jumping is restricted to tandem jumping, though if an individual develops diabetes after he/she has already been jumping, the case will be judged by the British Parachute Association on individual merits.

Motor racing

Insulin-treated diabetics are also banned from holding a competitive driving licence and so they cannot compete in motor racing.

Bobsleigh

It is unlikely that insulin-treated diabetics would be passed as bobsleigh drivers in the medical examinations that all potential competitors must have.

PARTICIPATION RESTRICTED

A number of sporting bodies impose certain restrictions upon people with diabetes; some of these are simply to satisfy insurance requirements, whereas some are designed to ascertain individual suitability to participate. The sports of sub-aqua diving and horse racing are good examples of how attitudes to people with diabetes are changing, and of how the regulations imposed by sports' governing bodies can be changed by the pressure of well balanced arguments and sound medical advice.

Sub-aqua diving

People with insulin-treated diabetes were at one time prevented from underwater swimming, but the regulations of the British Sub-Aqua Club were changed so that people with insulin-treated diabetes could dive, provided certain criteria could be fulfilled. A medical referee must certify the diver with diabetes as being fit and in good health. Their diving buddy should be someone who is either a regular diving partner and familiar with the problems that may be experienced by someone with diabetes or a trained medic or paramedic.

Horse racing

People on insulin are not permitted to become jockeys, but each case is examined individually. One of the authors has recently been a member of an independent panel of experts, which has advised the Jockey Club on the case of a prominent jockey who has recently developed diabetes. His case is being very sympathetically reviewed, with every hope that he will be allowed to continue to ride.

Ballooning

The British Balloon and Airship Club require a declaration of fitness to be completed and countersigned by the individual's own doctor, who is therefore completely empowered to decide on the fitness of an individual.

Canoeing

Although there are no restrictions on a person with diabetes canoeing, an individual with diabetes can be granted a coaching award only if they undergo annual medical review. A general practitioner or consultant must confirm that their diabetes is stable and undertakes to notify the British Canoe Union of any change in circumstance. If an existing coaching scheme member develops diabetes, they will be temporarily suspended pending stabilisation of diabetes.

Gliding

People with diabetes are allowed to fly as a glider pilot if a declaration of fitness is endorsed by a general practitioner or an authorised medical examiner, but should not expect to become instructors, enter competition or undertake long cross-country flights.

Motorcycling

Motorcycling is relatively open to people with diabetes. Participation in special events requires a medical certificate to be produced; the certificate asks if the participant has diabetes, but if the diabetes is stable and the subject is not subject to frequent hypos, they should be passed as fit to race. Medicals are required every 5 years. No medicals are required for trials, endurance, drag and sprint competitions, except at international level.

Rowing

Surprisingly, although there are no restrictions on membership of the Great Britain Rowing Team, the Amateur Rowing Association require insulin-treated diabetics to be under regular medical supervision; participation is allowed if glycaemic control is good and the subject is 'free of hypoglycaemic attacks'.

Powerboats

Individuals interested in power boat racing are assessed on the basis of previous sailing experience, glycaemic control and frequency of hypoglycaemia, but are likely to be passed fit to race if these parameters are deemed appropriate.

Triathlon

The British Triathlon Association imposes no restrictions upon people with diabetes, but insists that the fact that one has diabetes should be written on the back of the race number and that one of the medical professionals in attendance should be aware that the individual has diabetes.

The vast majority of sports are entirely open to people with diabetes and impose no restrictions upon participation. If in doubt, the national sport-governing body should be contacted; the British Diabetic Association will supply an up-to-date list of addresses of all sports' associations together with regulations and restrictions on request and we are grateful to them for much of the information contained in this chapter.

REFERENCES

1. Ainsworth BE, Haskell WL, Leon AS *et al.* Compendium of physical activities: classification of energy costs of human physical activities. *Med Sci Sports Exerc* 1993; **25:** 71–80
2. Quoted in *Balance* no. 164. 13–15 July/August 1998 British Diabetic Association Publications, London
3. Bergeron MF, Maresh CM, Kraemer WJ, Abraham A, Conroy B, Gabaree C. Tennis: physiological profile during match play. *Int J Sports Med* 1991; **12:** 474–479

8

Diabetes and the Marathon

BILL BURR

Pinderfields Hospital, Wakefield, UK

INTRODUCTION

The marathon represents a supreme athletic challenge, and for those runners who also happen to have diabetes the challenge is even more daunting. An individual with diabetes who is contemplating running a marathon should be fairly clear about the magnitude of the undertaking, and their reasons for attempting it. The extreme nature of the exertion, and the sustained training required over many months, demand enormous attention to detail, and will almost certainly cause problems with diabetic control.

There are many variables affecting diabetic control in relation to marathon running, and it is difficult to produce a single set of recommendations. People vary in physique and level of fitness as well as in athletic ability. On top of this, people with diabetes have additional variables related to such things as their treatment regimen and insulin type and dosage. They also vary in terms of the speed with which they become hyperglycaemic and develop ketones when insulin levels are inadequate. If an individual has absolutely no ability to secrete insulin, their insulin requirement is about 1 unit/kg body weight/day. They will tend to become hyperglycaemic quite rapidly when insulin deprived. People with lower insulin requirements have varying degrees of residual insulin secretion, and tend to be less prone

Exercise and Sport in Diabetes. Edited by Bill Burr and Dinesh Nagi.
© 1999 John Wiley & Sons Ltd.

to severe hyperglycaemia and ketosis. It may be somewhat easier for such an individual to maintain metabolic control during the severe physical stresses of the marathon than for someone with no residual insulin secretion. It follows that there will inevitably be a great deal of 'trial and error' before a particular individual discovers the precise adjustments to their diabetic routine which will enable them to train and compete safely and effectively in the marathon.

Some general guidelines will be given, and then a number of examples of how different individuals have put these into practice.

GUIDELINES

PRE-EXERCISE HEALTH CHECK

If you have not been in the habit of taking regular exercise, it would be wise to consult your general practitioner or hospital consultant to make sure there are no health reasons why you should avoid heavy exertion. The examination should include feet, eyes, heart and chest, and measurement of blood pressure. The urine should be checked for protein, and glycated haemoglobin (HbAlc) should be measured to check diabetic control. Depending on age and/or symptoms, it may be considered advisable to have an ECG or exercise test.

FOOTWEAR, CLOTHING, AND EQUIPMENT

Clothing should be comfortable; shorts need to have a pocket for dextrose tablets. A tracksuit is needed for cold weather only. Shoes are the most important item of equipment, especially for runs over about 4 miles. They need to be good quality, well fitting, and must be 'broken in' carefully during shorter runs, with a special check of the feet for any signs of blistering. They need thick, shock-absorbing soles, and in addition it is sensible to wear hosiery which has maximum cushioning ability (e.g., Thorlo®). When training, or even when competing, it may be useful to carry a 'bumbag' or small rucksack containing blood testing kit, identification, glucose tablets and drinks, contact numbers and advice for dealing with hypoglycaemia.

KEEPING IN CONTACT

It is wise to make sure that someone knows where you are going to be running, and what time you expect to return. This is important on dark evenings and on little-used roads, and is absolutely essential when running cross-country. However well prepared you are, there is going to be an increased risk of hypoglycaemia when running, and it is vital that help should be available when this happens. It is also important to wear some form of identification, such as an 'SOS' bracelet, to confirm the fact that you have diabetes and to give a contact number in case of emergency.

It is worth giving some thought to the idea of joining a local running club. This can provide a source of running partners, as well as providing advice on type and availability of equipment, and on loosening-up exercises.

DIARY

Mention has already been made of the 'trial and error' approach which is needed while you are tailoring your diet and insulin regimen to suit different training and competition schedules. The learning process is greatly helped if detailed records are kept—especially in the early stages. Ideally a log-book should contain details of:

- Distance run
- Time taken
- Blood glucose levels before and after run
- Timing, amount, and type of insulin before and after
- Timing, amount, and type of food taken 2–3 h before and up to 8 h after the run
- Time of day
- Weather conditions and an estimate of the effect these have on the intensity of effort
- Hypoglycaemia—timing, warning symptoms (e.g. weakness, blurred vision, feeling dizzy or maybe no warning), action taken
- General comments e.g. hypoglycaemia occurring 12 h afterwards, or overnight. Changes in fitness and running speed, changes in body weight (lower body weight will reduce insulin requirements). Ideas for future treatment adjustments

TRAINING

The golden rule is to build up gradually both the length and the intensity of training runs. Where you actually start from will depend on your general level of fitness, and on whether or not you are running or taking part in active sports on a regular basis. For instance, a sedentary, inactive person should begin by walking, and build up both speed and distance—e.g. $\frac{1}{2}$, 1, 2, 3 miles—before starting to jog. If you are regularly playing sport such as soccer, rugby, or squash you will probably be able to start by jogging 2–3 miles, and build up from this.

As the person with diabetes starts to do endurance training on a regular basis (say three training runs per week), there will be a progressive reduction in insulin requirements of between 25 and 40%. This is irrespective of any insulin reductions needed on the day of exercise, and is a reflection of the improved insulin sensitivity brought about by regular exercise. Most athletes find that this insulin sensitivity wears off within about a week when training stops.

DIABETIC CONTROL AND MONITORING

The need for good diabetic control before exercise has been stressed before (see Chapter 2). Ideally, the blood glucose should be between 6 and 10 mmol/l (110–180 mg/dl) at the start of exertion. If the glucose is above 14 mmol/l (250 mg/dl), the urine should be checked for ketones, and if they are present the session should be cancelled. Figure 8.1 shows how exercise can cause serious worsening of ketosis in an individual whose diabetes is out of control at the start of exercise.

As mentioned elsewhere, the physiological response in a non-diabetic to endurance events is to reduce insulin levels to a minimum, to allow release of glucose from the liver, and to make sure that glucose uptake by muscles is not excessive. The person with diabetes has to try to mimic this situation by reducing insulin doses, but without becoming deficient in insulin to the point of allowing ketoacidosis to occur.

Blood glucose will need to be checked 15–30 min before training or competing, as mentioned above. If it is below 6 mmol/l, extra carbohydrate in the form of a chocolate bar or high-carbohydrate drink is needed. Some athletes have recommended testing blood glucose hourly throughout the marathon, but this would seem excessive for most people, and is perhaps feasible only during training runs.

After running, it is necessary to check blood glucose after 30 min or so, to guide the amount of carbohydrate replacement required.

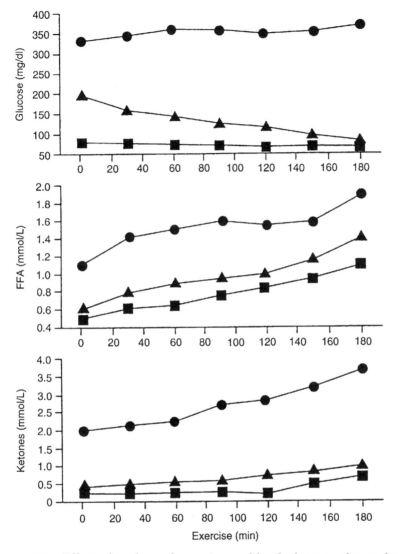

Figure 8.1. Effect of prolonged exercise on blood glucose, plasma ketone bodies (acetoacetate and β-hydroxybutyrate) and plasma free fatty acids (FFA) in healthy control participants (■), diabetic patients in moderate control (▲) and ketotic diabetic patients (●). Adapted from Berger M, *et al.*, *Diabetologia* 1977; 13: 355–365 by permission.

Monitoring can revert to normal after this, with the exception that it is absolutely vital to check blood glucose before bed to try to avoid overnight hypoglycaemia.

INSULIN DOSE

It is really difficult to generalise about the extent of insulin dose reductions for the marathon. The simplest situation is that of someone on treatment with a continuous subcutaneous insulin infusion. These people find that the basal infusion rate needs to be reduced by 50% or more, and additional carbohydrate may still have to be taken during the event. For people on treatment with infused soluble insulin (e.g. Actrapid or Humulin S), the infusion rate needs to be reduced 30 min *before* the race. If the insulin analogue Humalog (lispro insulin) is being infused, the rate can be reduced immediately before the event because of the rapid absorption of subcutaneous Humalog.

The most common insulin regimen in Europe is the so-called 'basal/bolus' regimen, in which a bedtime dose of isophane, lente or ultralente insulin is taken together with pre-prandial soluble insulin or Humalog. On this type of treatment schedule, most athletes would take the normal dose of insulin on the night before the marathon, or would make only a slight reduction (10%). They would make variable and at times radical reductions in the preprandial dose before the event. The range of dose reduction ranges from about 20% to 90%, and one of the major factors determining the size of the reduction is the amount of planned carbohydrate intake during the race (see below). The timing of the soluble insulin injection before a race is critical. It is important that the insulin levels are declining before starting sustained exercise, and this means that the injection of soluble insulin should be about 90–120 min before the race, while Humalog should be taken about 60 min before the event.

One other insulin regimen which is still quite commonly encountered is that in which there is a twice-daily injection of a mixture of soluble and isophane or lente insulins. It is probably better for an athlete to be using free mixtures of short- and intermediate-acting insulins rather than pre-mixed insulins, since this allows a greater degree of flexibility in adjusting doses to cope with training and competitions. For races taking place in the morning, the reductions in short-acting insulin would be similar to those made on a basal/bolus regimen, together with a modest reduction in intermediate insulin (about 20%). For races in the afternoon, the morning short-acting insulin would not be altered, but the intermediate insulin would be drastically reduced or omitted.

After the race, people again have differing approaches to making adjustments to their insulin dose. Many athletes take quite large amounts of freely absorbed carbohydrate 30–60 min after the race, and if so they would take either the usual insulin to cover this or would make a modest reduction. Later in the day and overnight, and even through the next day, there is going to be a strong tendency to develop delayed hypoglycaemia, which has to be countered by extra carbohydrate intake and reduced insulin. The reasons for this have been explained elsewhere (Chapter 2) but, in simple terms, sustained exercise has a dramatic and prolonged (12–24 h or more) effect on muscle sensitivity to insulin. More glucose is removed from the bloodstream for a given amount of insulin. Muscle glycogen stores are being replenished during this time, and this increases the demand for blood glucose (Chapter 1). It is reasonable to reduce the bedtime insulin on a basal/bolus regimen by 20% or so, and to make a similar reduction to the teatime intermediate insulin for those on twice-daily injections, and to combine this with a substantial increase in evening carbohydrate intake.

FOOD AND FLUID INTAKE

General dietary guidelines for those taking part in demanding athletic events, involving sustained, high-intensity effort, are summarised in Table 8.1.

Advice specifically relating to the marathon is given below.

Several Days Pre-event

Before undertaking a major endurance event such as the marathon, it is customary to phase-down training in the week before the event, and to increase carbohydrate intake to 70% or more of the calorie intake. For those with diabetes, this advice would seem to hold true, but for the purposes of so-called 'carbo-loading', it would be wise to stick to foods with a low glycaemic index (see Chapter 1). These

Table 8.1. Summary of dietary recommendations for elite athletes

Four days before competition;
- Taper training
- Carbohydrate loading: 8–10 g/kg body mass per day for 3–4 days

Before competition:
- 3–4 h before competition, eat easily digestible high carbohydrate meal, 1–2 g/kg body mass
- For competitors who have diabetes, this meal should consist of carbohydrates with a low glycaemic index
- Avoid concentrated (> 8% glucose) glucose drinks within an hour of exercise (risk of gastrointestinal discomfort)

During exercise:
- Carbohydrate/electrolyte solutions are helpful and delay glycogen depletion and avoid dehydration
- Suitable sports drinks should be consumed at the rate of 120–150 ml for every 15 min of exercise

During recovery from exercise:
- 50 g carbohydrate immediately after exercise and 8–10 g carbohydrate/kg body weight in 24 h. High-glycaemic-index foods in the first 6 h, and continued for the 24 h when rapid recovery is needed
- Athletes with diabetes should avoid high-glycaemic-index foods, except in the immediate post-exercise period
- Addition of protein may speed recovery of glycogen stores

carbohydrate foods are complex, require digestion to take place before absorption of simple sugars can occur, and therefore have the least effect on blood glucose and insulin requirements. The recommended daily intake of carbohydrate for those who do not have diabetes is 8–10 g/kg body weight for 3 or 4 days before the race, and there is no reason why this advice should not apply also for those with diabetes.

Pre-exercise meals

Most people with diabetes feel that it is important to have a substantial, high-carbohydrate meal before the competition. This advice has been summed up as 'It's important to have ballast in the hold'. The drawback is that many people feel uncomfortable or are prone to stomach cramps if they eat excessively before exercise. As a compromise, the pre-marathon meal should be taken about 2 h before the event for those using ordinary soluble insulin. For those using Humalog, 1–1.5 h before the race would be appropriate. For this meal, it would be sensible to use mainly carbohydrate with a low glycaemic index. The amount to be taken will be governed by trial and error, according to the amount that can comfortably be eaten. As a guide, it would be reasonable to aim for 2–4 g of carbohydrate per kg body weight.

Pre-exercise Drinks

As mentioned in Chapter 1, ingestion of high-carbohydrate (25% or more) drinks before a race is not recommended because of the tendency to cause delayed stomach emptying and gastrointestinal disturbance. Commercially available carbohydrate–electrolyte solutions contain 5–8% carbohydrate, and do not cause delayed stomach emptying or abdominal cramps. It is reasonable to use these immediately before the race, especially if there is a need to correct relative hypoglycaemia at this time (blood glucose < 6 mmol/l). It should be possible to drink 500 ml of these solutions without detriment to athletic performance.

Carbohydrate Intake During the Race

It is important to take regular fluid throughout the race to prevent dehydration, and this fluid should be taken regularly according to a fixed plan, without waiting for the development of thirst. Carbohydrate–electrolyte drinks have been developed commercially for just this type of situation, and have been found to be well tolerated. Chapter 1 summed up evidence to show that taking these solutions regularly through prolonged exercise has a glycogen-sparing action which delays the onset of exhaustion. People with diabetes may also benefit from taking these drinks, although it will be necessary to experiment during long-distance training runs to discover how much can be taken without producing hyperglycaemia. The prevailing levels of blood insulin will be a major determining factor, but it is also true that actively contracting muscles are remarkably able to dispose of blood glucose in the presence of very low levels of insulin.

If you have successfully reduced your insulin you may have no need to take additional carbohydrate during the race, and many athletes with diabetes prefer to run the whole distance with virtually no additional carbohydrate. Others prefer to take additional food in the form of bananas, cereal bars or chocolate.

Carbohydrate and Food Intake after Exercise

Very rapid recovery from exercise is only strictly relevant to athletes who are taking part in events which require daily performance for days or weeks. There is evidence that restoration of muscle glycogen levels and exercise capacity can be speeded by taking high-glycaemic-index carbohydrates, and by increasing daily carbohydrate intake by 50% (from 6 g/kg body to 9 g/kg body weight/day). For the 'ordinary' marathon runner with diabetes, it is probably sufficient to replace carbohydrate and fluid immediately after the event using carbohydrate–electrolyte solutions. Later in the day it would be wise to take a large meal consisting mainly of low-glycaemic-index carbohydrate to assist the replenishment of glycogen stores overnight. Even with reductions of insulin dose and extra carbohydrate, there will still be a tendency to hypoglycaemia on the following morning, requiring extra carbohydrate and reduced insulin. Some athletes report that this effect can continue for 48 h.

PERSONAL VIEWS

DAWN KENWRIGHT

Dawn was already an international athlete when she developed type 1 diabetes in 1993, at the age of 37. She specialised in mountain and cross-country running. She was hospitalised to commence insulin treatment, but started running again within 3 days of discharge, actually competed 3 weeks after this, and ran in an international after 6 weeks!

She attributes her success to great determination and discipline in taking four injections of insulin daily and monitoring and recording blood sugars regularly, as well as controlling diet and mealtimes. She runs a lot on her own, and stresses the need to carry identification, to let people know of her whereabouts, and to carry adequate supplies of glucose.

Dawn's insulin regimen consists of human soluble insulin 4, 4, and 6 units before breakfast, lunch and evening meal respectively, and 8 units of human isophane at night. She monitors blood glucose before and after every run, and sometimes during runs when not competing. She reduces her soluble insulin before major events, and takes large amounts of complex carbohydrate during the build-up. During an event, she finds that she is unable to eat carbohydrate, and she also cannot tolerate isotonic drinks. She has managed to run for 5 h at high altitude without taking carbohydrate. She takes complex carbohydrate soon after the run, and has a marked tendency to delayed hypoglycaemia 24 or even 48 h after the event.

MATTHEW KILN

Dr Matthew Kiln is a general practitioner, who has run more than 12 marathons. He has type 1 diabetes, which is controlled by twice-daily injections of a mixture of soluble and lente insulins. He uses beef insulins, having experienced problems with hypoglycaemia while taking human insulin.

During training runs of up to 15 miles, Matthew prefers to take his usual insulin dose while maintaining his blood glucose with frequent carbohydrates. At times he has found difficulties in taking adequate carbohydrate without feeling sick, because by trial and error he has established that he needs about 7–12 g of carbohydrate per mile. This varies according to the time of day, and is presumably related to the level of free insulin circulating during the run.

For the marathon itself Matthew switches his approach, and takes a drastically reduced dose of soluble insulin only on the morning of the race, taking for instance just two units of soluble insulin instead of his usual 4 units soluble and 14 units lente. With this low dose, and taking 30 g of carbohydrate during the race, he began with a blood sugar of 7 mmol/l, and finished with a blood glucose of 4 mmol/l.

SUMMARY

Even though running the marathon is a supreme athletic challenge, many people with diabetes have successfully attempted it with levels of competence ranging from 'fun' running in the London Marathon to international competition.

It is undoubtedly a serious undertaking, which requires great commitment. There are many benefits from taking part, including the pride of achievement as well as increased self knowledge and understanding of diabetes.

FURTHER READING

a. Kibirige M, Court S. *Childhood and Adolescent Diabetes*. In: Court, S & Lamb WH, eds. *Exercise and Diabetes*, p. 273–288. John Wiley & Sons, Chichester, 1997.
b. Ruderman N, Devlin JT (eds) *The Health Professional's Guide to Diabetes and Exercise*. American Diabetes Association, Alexandria 1995.
c. Williams C, Devlin JT (eds). *Foods, Nutrition and Sports Performance*. E & FN Spon, London, 1992.
d. Young JC. Exercise prescription for individuals with metabolic disorders. *Sports Med* 1995. **1**: 43–54.

USEFUL ADDRESSES

1. American Diabetes Association
   National Service Center
   1660 Duke Street
   Alexandria
   Virginia 22314
   USA

2. British Diabetic Association
   10 Queen Anne Street
   London
   W1M 0BD
   UK
   BDA Careline; Telephone: 0171-636-6112

3. The International Diabetic Athletes Association
   1647-B West Bethany Home Road
   Phoenix
   Arizona 85015
   USA
   e-mail: idaa@diabetes-exercise.org
   website: http://www.diabetes-exercise.org

4. The National Sports Institute
   c/o St Bartholomew's Medical College
   Charterhouse Square
   London
   EC1M 6BQ
   UK

9

Adoption and Maintenance of a Physical Activity Programme for People with Diabetes

ELIZABETH MARSDEN

Canterbury Christ Church University College, Canterbury, UK

TRADITIONAL ATTITUDES AND VIEWS ABOUT EXERCISE

The benefits of regular exercise for people with diabetes have been outlined in Chapter 4. During recent years, Diabetes health professionals, the World Health Organization[1], various books, journals, and magazines have promoted the idea that regular exercise should be undertaken by people with diabetes if they are to stay healthy and fit. The traditional exercise prescription for both health gains and physical fitness benefits has been based on guidelines by the American College of Sports Medicine, first produced in 1978 and reviewed again in 1990[2]. These guidelines stated that a minimum of at least three 20 min sessions per week of vigorous-intensity exercise (60–85% maximum heart rate) should be undertaken.

The word 'exercise' has certain connotations and evokes strongly held views amongst both patients and health professionals[3]. The traditional view has been that, in order to do any good, exercise must be 'hard' and, therefore, an activity in which only younger

Exercise and Sport in Diabetes. Edited by Bill Burr and Dinesh Nagi.

people were likely to engage. A large number of men and women have also been deterred by popular images of sport and exercise, as they do not consider themselves to be 'sporty types'[4]. A survey of West of Scotland diabetes clinics was carried out to establish the percentage of regular exercisers amongst the insulin dependent population, and showed that only 28% regarded themselves as regular exercisers, compared with 41% of NHS staff and 32% of Further Education College students[5]. At present, there is little information to show what proportion of people with type 2 diabetes are taking regular exercise, but it is likely to be less than the 25% or so reported from surveys of the general population[6,7]. It appears that beginning and 'staying with' a physical activity programme is difficult for most people, and especially those with diabetes.

MODERN THINKING ABOUT EXERCISE

Early views concerning the health benefits of exercise, such as that from the American Heart Association in 1992[8], were focussed on obtaining a training effect for fitness. They recommended activity intensities exceeding 60% of maximum heart rate to lower lipids and control diabetes and obesity. These levels of activity are likely to be inappropriate and unrealistic for a sedentary population and may partly account for high drop-out rates and poor compliance. Fortunately, there is now ample evidence that low-to-moderate-intensity activities performed regularly and frequently may have long-term health benefits and lower the risk of cardiovascular disease[9-11]. The Centre for Disease Control in the USA highlighted that health benefits could be gained from encouraging people to embark on moderate-intensity activities such as walking, stair climbing and household chores and that the physical activity can be built up throughout the day[12]. It is, therefore, necessary to re-examine the information given to sedentary people with diabetes regarding exercise and physical activity. A strategy for encouraging people with diabetes to take up physical activity is more likely to succeed if the message is aimed at goals and activities that are desirable and also attainable by this population.

ESSENTIAL ATTRIBUTES OF A PHYSICAL ACTIVITY PROGRAMME FOR PEOPLE WITH DIABETES

The relationship between the terms 'physical fitness', 'exercise' and 'physical activity' can be understood from the following definitions by Caspersen, Powell and Christenson[13].

> Exercise is a planned, structured and repetitive bodily movement done to improve or maintain one or more components of physical fitness. Physical activity is any bodily movement produced by skeletal muscle that results in energy expenditure.

A good exercise and physical activity programme share basic ingredients. Although the intensity of an exercise programme in order to enhance fitness is necessarily higher, both should result in health benefits[14]. A balanced programme, containing components of flexibility, aerobic and muscular endurance work, is desirable. Programmes may also contain speed and muscular strength work for those involved in specific sports which require training in these components.

FLEXIBILITY

Insufficient attention is paid to flexibility as most believe it to be relatively unimportant. Inflexible joints, particularly in older people, can cause a great deal of difficulty in performing ordinary daily tasks such as getting out of a chair or even crossing a road before the 'green man' turns red! Good flexibility is the ability to move joints comfortably through their whole range, thus allowing smooth and effective movements in sporting activities and daily tasks. It also helps to prevent injury from muscle pulls. Flexibility, like the other components of a good programme, will be lost during periods of inactivity and should, therefore, be regularly practised.

AEROBIC CAPACITY

The aerobic component of a physical activity programme is important, especially for people with diabetes, as it challenges the cardiovascular system. Cardiovascular problems are of major concern in diabetic complications and there is now much evidence to show the protective value of aerobic exercise to the cardiovascular system[15–17].

STRENGTH

Strength training may be designed either to lift the maximum weight in a single effort (muscular strength) or to lift submaximal loads for a longer period of time (muscular endurance). Muscular endurance is more important for most sporting activities, to carry out everyday tasks comfortably and even to maintain a pain-free upright posture. A balanced exercise or physical activity programme should contain each of the three most important components: flexibility, aerobic component, and muscular endurance.

PREPARATION FOR EXERCISE

READY TO START?

Before embarking on an activity programme, the sedentary person with diabetes will need support in several ways. Firstly, a basic understanding of how exercise will affect his/her treatment and daily diabetes management is essential. This will require professional advice, which is unlikely to be achieved in the context of a busy routine diabetes clinic: it will need a specific appointment with the person responsible for giving exercise advice in the clinic. The advice given should include a brief summary of the known benefits, risks, and type of physical activity suitable for this individual. Insulin-treated patients will need detailed instruction for monitoring blood sugar and adjusting food and insulin in relation to exercise (see Chapter 2). The professional giving this advice should have a detailed knowledge of associated conditions such as heart disease and specific complications of diabetes which are relevant to increasing physical activity. Formal exercise testing (on a treadmill) as a preliminary check before entering an exercise/activity programme is rarely thought to be necessary in UK clinics, and any risks are considered to be slight as long as there is a gradual build-up of physical activity with instructions to report any problems.

BEST FOOT FORWARD...

Once the would-be exerciser has been given medical approval and has a sound understanding of the effects of physical exercise, she or he will require a degree of patience in starting slowly and comfortably. Physical activity can be of value only if it becomes a regular part of someone's life. Aiming too high at the start is likely to result in discomfort, injury or ill health and therefore disappointment, frustration and poor compliance. To avoid these early setbacks, a low-intensity activity at the outset and gradual build-up of activity is strongly recommended.

The next stage of preparation for exercise/activity is to consider the usual lifestyle and to estimate whether it will be easier to accommodate small bouts of physical activity, which will add up to 30–60 min per day, or whether specific exercise sessions several times a week are easier to fit into what is probably already a busy schedule. Whatever decision is made, each session should include flexibility, aerobic activity and muscular endurance. It is also important to decide whether the aim of an exercise programme is to gain fitness and health benefits or health benefits alone. If both fitness and health benefits are required then a target heart rate of between 65–85% of maximum for about 20 min per session and at least three times per week should be the aim. Using Borg's 'Rate of Perceived Exertion' (RPE) chart (Table 9.1)[18], this normally means that an exerciser is working at between level 13 and 15. It may be helpful to have a baseline fitness test at a gym or human performance laboratory. The instructor will be able to advise at what level to start and when to return for a follow-up test which will show whether the exercise programme is working for increased fitness. It is currently not known what level of activity is required for health benefits alone, as the 'dose–response' equation is complex[19]. However, since it is recognised that keeping sedentary people active is extremely important for their health, working at a comfortable level of intensity is the best rule of thumb—i.e. between 11 and 13 on the RPE scale and up to 60% of maximum heart rate. For some people with diabetes even moderate-intensity activity will be impossible, and the basic rule must be that any increase in physical activity is desirable, and goals need to be set accordingly.

Table 9.1. Borg Perceived Exertion Scale

Rating of perceived exertion (RPE)	Verbal description of RPE
6	
7	Very, very light
8	
9	Very light
10	
11	Fairly light
12	
13	Somewhat hard
14	
15	Hard
16	
17	Very hard
18	
19	Very, very hard
20	

From reference 18, by permission of The American College of Sports Medicine.

...AND OFF WE GO

Warm-up

Any period of activity should ideally begin with a warm-up period. The importance of warming up is based on sound physiological principles. During warm-up the temperature of the large muscle groups is increased, which allows increased force and velocity of muscular contraction as well as increased blood and oxygen supply to the fibres. Chemical reactions within the muscle tissue are increased, and energy for muscle contraction is increased. Finally, the warm-up helps prevent tears and damage to connective tissue and thereby prevents joint injury. Warm-up for a beginner should be at least 10 min, and should consist of extremely light, large muscle group activity such as walking, easy jogging and swinging movements.

If warm-up is too short or omitted, within the first few minutes of starting the main exercise session the exerciser will feel discomfort, rapid heart rate, heavy breathing and muscle fatigue due to the body's inability to use its aerobic system and its dependence on the anaerobic system.

Flexibility exercises

Once warm-up is completed, the beginning exerciser is advised to engage in some flexibility practice of the large muscle groups. Modern stretching techniques are designed to produce slow and gradual lengthening of the muscles with the full stretch being held for 15–30 s. Muscles stretched in this way are also relaxed. There are many different kinds of stretching exercises: Appendix 1 illustrates a selection of sequential stretches beginning with the large group of leg muscles, moving onto muscles of the trunk, and finally stretches of the arms and shoulders.

Aerobic exercises

Essentially, aerobic activity is rhythmic, repetitive and causes the muscles to work at a level where they require oxygen for the release of energy. There is a wide selection of activities suitable for the aerobic component of an exercise or physical activity programme. It is best to select those which are appropriate to the individual's needs and which are enjoyable. If, for example, the beginning exerciser is overweight, she or he may feel very uncomfortable performing high-impact or jarring activities such as jogging or work with a skipping rope. He or she may also feel ill at ease in a class situation where skimpy and tight clothing is the norm. However, the same individual may feel relaxed and comfortable using a bicycle, rowing machine or walking briskly. A regular exerciser may choose a mixture of swimming, playing football, canoeing or jogging for his/her programme. Examples of aerobic exercise include brisk walking, cycling, cross-country skiing, hillwalking, canoeing, rowing, jogging, swimming and any running game. As muscles, including the heart muscles, become conditioned to activity, it is possible and desirable to work for longer or to increase the intensity over a period of weeks or months.

The intensity of exercise for a training effect can be calculated from the heart rate: '220 minus the age' will give an estimate of maximum heart rate in beats per minute. In order for fitness to be improved, the pulse rate should be between 65% and 85% of maximum heart rate. It is wise to calculate what the heart rate should be for a 10 or 15 second count as this is easy to take during the exercise session. For example, a 45-year-old woman who enjoys cycling has decided to enter a cycle marathon. She would like to target her training programme towards becoming fitter. Using the calculation to find her estimated maximum heart rate ($220 - 45 = 175$ beats per minute), she can work out that in order to be training hard enough she will need to cycle so that her heart rate is raised to between 65% and 85% of 175; i.e. between 114 and 149 beats per minute. If gaining fitness is not as important as gaining health benefits, then the target heart rate may be only between 50% and 60% of the maximum heart rate. The perceived exertion chart described earlier (Table 9.1) is also useful in determining the correct intensity for an individual.

Muscular endurance

Muscular endurance activities also play an important part in the complete exercise or physical activity programme. Without a degree of muscular endurance, simple tasks such as gardening, housework or changing a car tyre can become difficult and may result in injury or muscle strain. There are several training principles that should be understood before embarking on the muscular endurance part of the training programme.

In order to improve muscular endurance, the principle of progressive overload must be applied. The beginning exerciser will be unfamiliar with the load values which he/she is capable of lifting, so it is best to start with fairly light weights. The number of repetitions performed (i.e. how many times the same exercise is repeated) is normally around 12 to induce endurance. At the correct load, the individual will find repetitions 10, 11 and 12 hard to complete but still manageable. At the beginning of an exercise programme, it is best to limit the number of sets of repetitions to one or two to avoid muscle soreness. As the exerciser becomes more able, and muscles become used to endurance, another set of 12 repetitions can be added to the programme. Eventually, a full three sets can be performed regularly.

A complete muscular endurance programme will include a wide variety of different types of exercises so that a balance is achieved. Often a person's own body weight serves well as the load in the exercise. Muscular endurance improves in those muscles that are specifically being trained. Most exercisers like to vary their programme for muscular endurance quite frequently and the illustrations given in Appendix 2 offer some examples of those exercises that will result in an all-over body conditioning programme. These have been chosen because no special equipment is required and they can be done anywhere. Exercises can be made progressively more difficult by increasing the level or by increasing the repetitions. It is important to work all of the large muscle groups in any one programme.

Cooling down

Once the physical activity session is completed, it is necessary to spend a few minutes in cooling down. If the body goes from a state of pumping blood at a much increased rate to stopping suddenly, dizziness, nausea or light-headedness may be experienced. The working muscles push blood back to the heart but when they stop suddenly without a period of cooling down the blood pools in the muscles instead of being forced back to the heart. A transition period is required for transferring from hard muscular work to light muscular work. Cooling down is as important as warming up.

Berg[20] maintained that a good aerobic component leaves the exerciser feeling more energetic, vitalised, relaxed and happy after the exercise than before. If varied and enjoyable types of exercise have been chosen and the sessions have been easily accommodated into the individual's lifestyle, then anxiety and stress are lessened—which in turn has a beneficial effect on a person's well-being and quality of life. Self-esteem and feelings of achievement add to the 'feel good' effect. In subjects with diabetes, these benefits may also have a positive impact on blood glucose control and the feeling of well-being and self-reliance may engage these individuals into taking a more active role in management of their diabetes.

Choosing how to fit exercise or periods of physical activity into an already busy life does take a great deal of thought and planning. In order to gain either health or fitness benefits, exercise and physical activity must be performed on a regular basis. It may be easier for people with diabetes to achieve a better blood glucose balance when each day's energy expenditure is relatively stable[20], but the sedentary individual who decides to aim for health benefits by taking short bursts of physical activity adding up to 30 min per day should remember that a complete programme includes muscular endurance, aerobic and flexibility components. It is likely that the short bursts of physical activity throughout the day will be largely aerobic in nature and provision needs to be made to include some muscular endurance and flexibility components at other times during the week. One of the most difficult problems in exercise and physical activity programmes is to find ways to 'stay with' physical activity—i.e. to increase long-term compliance.

CHANGING BEHAVIOUR

BEHAVIOUR MODIFICATION IN RELATION TO EXERCISE

Sallis and Hovell[21] proposed a framework for studying exercise behaviour. The four main stages are shown in Figure 9.1.

This model highlights the fact that exercise adoption is a dynamic process. Twelve years earlier, Prochaska[22] proposed a transtheoretical

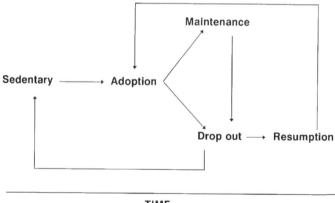

Figure 9.1. Four major phases of the natural history of exercise. From reference 21, by permission of *Exercise and Sports Science Review*

model of behaviour change ('Stages of Change' model), believing that behaviour at any one time can be identified on a spectrum with clearly defined stages.

Stage theory lies between that of traits and states, in which traits are considered to be stable and unchanging and states are relatively unstable and changeable with time. Stages may be stable for long periods of time but are always open to change[23]. These stages are considered in 6-monthly time periods as researchers have found that this is the optimum period that most subjects are prepared to contemplate. The stages of change (see Figure 9.2) are known as 'precontemplation' (no intention to change); 'contemplation' (actively thinking of changing a behaviour, considering pro and cons); 'preparation' (currently exercising, but not regularly); 'action' (currently exercising regularly but have only just started); 'maintenance' (change has taken place).

It is important to realise that the progression from one stage to another is not always linear, and that subjects frequently relapse to the precontemplation stage or from one stage to another. It is also well known that individuals may have to make several attempts through these stages of change before a behaviour change is firmly established.

The transtheoretical model described above helps both prediction and explanation of different people's behaviour towards health-related activities. Prochaska and DiClemente[24] originally used the model in their work on cessation of smoking but more recently[23] have

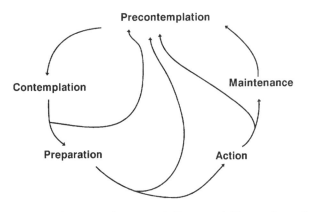

Figure 9.2. The transtheoretical (States of Change) model

applied this model to physical activity. They have targeted intervention strategies at the 'contemplator' and 'preparer' groups since these subjects are actually thinking about becoming regular exercisers. Although giving up smoking is relinquishing a negative health behaviour, and adoption of physical activity a positive one, there are a number of similarities, particularly if adoption of physical activity is viewed as giving up an inactive lifestyle. Marcus and Bess *et al.*[25,26] showed that a staged, matched, intervention based on this model was likely to be more successful in getting subjects to move from one stage to another. In a community-based intervention study, Marcus *et al.* used an intervention based on the stages of change model to increase physical activity in 610 subjects. They found that at baseline 39% of subjects were in contemplation, 37% in preparation and 24% were in action stage. Intervention consisted of three different sets of self-help materials, a resource manual describing physical activity, weekly fun walks, and activity nights. A stratified (by baseline stage) random sample of participants ($n = 236$) were contacted after intervention. The results of this reassessment showed that after 6 weeks of intervention 17% were now in contemplation, 24% were in preparation and 59% were in action stage. The results were encouraging in that the proportion of subjects in action phase doubled over the baseline evaluation. This was not a randomised intervention study, but the results suggest that such innovative exercise interventions may turn out to be successful in increasing the uptake of physical activity.

APPLICATION OF BEHAVIOUR MODIFICATION THEORY TO ADOPTION AND MAINTENANCE OF PHYSICAL ACTIVITY

The most recent national fitness survey[7] confirmed that participation rates in physical activity are low. The drop-out rate within 6 months of starting to exercise is over 50%, even amongst those clinical populations with the most to gain from regular physical activity[27]. Researchers have tried for many years to find successful intervention strategies to keep people active and admit: 'It is chastening to see yet again how little we understand of the zone between people's knowledge, attitudes and beliefs and their actual behaviour.'[28]

The Health Education Authority[29] has suggested that the Stages of Change (transtheoretical model) may be most useful for health care professionals to use because it is now possible to identify at which stage of change the patient is on the model's spectrum (Figure 9.2). This, in turn, would allow different strategies to be adopted for that particular stage in order to encourage exercise adoption and maintenance.

Using the Stages of Change model to assist in the adoption and maintenance of exercise behaviour

Referring a patient to an exercise class or prescribing an exercise programme (i.e. action), if he or she is in the pre-contemplation stage would be unlikely to be successful, and would be a waste of valuable time and resources. At this stage, it is best to present information about the risks of inactivity to this person, but not to push her/him any further at this point. Provision of important information such as the fact that the risk of suffering a cardiovascular event is much higher in a non-active person with diabetes, and that this risk is lower in those who take regular physical activity, may be sufficient incentive for a pre-contemplator to at least think about becoming active. It will also be helpful if pre-contemplators are made aware that should they wish to become more active in the future, they will have access to adequate support from the exercise counsellor or the person in the team who is taking responsibility for the promotion of exercise.

Contemplators and Preparers are likely to gain the most value from an exercise consultation as they are in the 'ready' stage. It would be helpful to find out the motivating factors and barriers to being physically active which are the most important to these individuals. Then, together, the counsellor and the would-be-regular exerciser can formulate a plan of action. Marsden[3] discovered that in subjects with diabetes the barriers to an increase in physical activity were not diabetes-specific (i.e. fear of having a hypo), but similar to those observed in non-diabetic subjects (i.e. 'not enough time', 'other hobbies come first', 'too lazy' and 'no-one with whom to exercise'). It is important to emphasise that the traditional view that physical activity must be of high intensity in order to gain any benefits, is not true. The term 'exercise' is often associated with high-intensity activity, which may strike fear into the hearts of would-be exercisers, who picture only lycra leotards or marathon runners' vests along with much sweating and discomfort. It may be better to stick to the term 'activity', and avoid the possibly negative connotations of the term 'exercise'.

Trying to find the contemplator's perceived barriers to activity is very important at this stage. It is also vital that the exercise counsellor listens to what the person with diabetes is saying and does not presume knowledge about an individual's feelings. Most health professionals have wrongly presumed that the fear of having a hypoglycaemic event whilst exercising is the biggest barrier: while it may be the health professional's biggest worry, it is not a major barrier to the patient with diabetes[3].

The main motivation for beginning physical activity is likely to be a desire to stay well, and to try to improve diabetic control and possibly prevent or delay diabetic complications[3]. People with diabetes, like any other population, also want to feel good and to have fun. In addition, some patients may not realise that there are positive psychological benefits to be gained, such as self-confidence, lack of anxiety and feelings of well-being. Biddle and Mutrie[30] have suggested that motivations may change over a person's lifespan and there is also evidence to suggest different motivating factors between men and women. Young men have been recorded as being more highly motivated to exercise if they gain social recognition, challenge and competition by doing so; young women, on the other hand, were seeking weight control, enjoyment and physical fitness. Ashford and Biddle[31] surveyed community sports centres' participants' reasons for undertaking physical activity and found that the older participants were looking for relaxation, social benefits and health benefits. The younger subjects were motivated by challenge and skill learning. Other researchers have found important motivating factors to be: improved health[32]; personality of class leader[33]; weight control[34]; to get fitter, to socialise and to feel better[7]; and 'medical advice'[35]. The latter point has been disputed by other researchers such as Shephard[36], who found that the patients in his research analysis rarely mentioned 'because the doctor told me to . . .' as a reason for beginning an exercise programme. It may suggest that the patients were not being advised by their doctor to exercise as part of a healthy lifestyle.

Those classing themselves as being either in the action or maintenance position on the spectrum should receive praise and every possible encouragement to continue. They may require help with short-, medium- and long-term goal setting or with planning some kind of reward for themselves to 'stay with' their programme. They may also require assurance that their activity level is correct for health benefits.

Relapsers are those people who have been active in the past but for whatever reason have ceased to be so. Many people will fall into this category at some point in their lives. It is important that they are not allowed to feel failures but to recognise that being a relapser is common and just one point on the stages of change spectrum. It may be helpful to remind them of the benefits that they enjoyed when they were active, and then to counsel them in the same way as contemplators if they are showing signs of wishing to be active again.

The necessity of including an exercise/physical activity advisor in the diabetes team

Diabetes-related interventions concerning physical activity have traditionally been in the form of information giving, occasionally providing fitness testing or, most recently, exercise and physical activity consultation. These important issues are rarely dealt with in a systematic way in most UK diabetes centres at present, and whether such advice is provided at all depends on the interests of members of the local diabetes team. Loughlan and Mutrie[37] found that exercise consultation was the most successful intervention, and the Health Education Authority[29] actively encourages primary health care teams to use consultation to promote exercise/physical activity whenever possible. An experienced counsellor is required to use the Stages of Change model as an instrument of intervention, working one-to-one with each patient. In view of the burgeoning numbers of patients with type 2 diabetes, in whom physical inactivity is probably the most important predisposing factor, and in whom the promotion of physical activity is fundamental to treatment (see Chapters 4 and 5), a full-time exercise adviser would be justified as a member of all diabetes teams.

Organising an Exercise Consultation Session

It is important that the health professional chosen to encourage physical activity amongst people with diabetes is a good listener. Whilst one aspect of the health professional's role is to provide exercise information, advice and encouragement, the skill of hearing what the patient says about his/her own situation, fears, problems, aspirations and goals is of utmost importance. Having first established where the patient fits on the Stages of Change model the following issues are helpful to consider during the exercise consultation.

Knowledge of the effects of bouts of physical activity upon the patient's diabetes is of prime importance. This knowledge should be given in a simple and easily understandable form, beginning with basic principles and building up to more detailed help, adjusting insulin levels etc., once she/he reaches a stage where exercise is more intense and/or prolonged.

For patients with type 2 diabetes, knowledge about the effects of exercise on diabetes can be combined with education about the importance of physical activity in controlling the disease, and preventing complications.

Starting to become active from a sedentary status may be far easier than the patient realises. It is useful to make a list of the things the patient does in one day—e.g. walks the dog, catches the bus to work, sits at a desk all day, catches the bus home and watches TV before walking the dog again. Next it is helpful to suggest how to increase the activity level in each of those areas—e.g. can he get off the bus one stop earlier on the way home and walk for an extra 5 minutes? Can he make sure he climbs at least one flight of stairs during the lunch break instead of taking the lift to the cafe? Can he walk the dog one block further? By working with the patient's already established lifestyle, extra physical activity can be added slowly and gradually. This technique is particularly useful in those with already busy time schedules. Encouraging a patient to do his or her normal activities with a little more effort is also beneficial—e.g. wash the car by hand rather than using a car wash.

Barriers preventing and motivations towards physical activity are very important for each person to consider and it may be helpful for patients to actually write down what benefits they think they will gain by becoming more active and what things are stopping them. These can be turned into reinforcement strategies and goals. The most common barriers are those concerned with lack of time, not having anyone to exercise with, not enjoying the thought of sweating and feeling uncomfortable and not being a sporty type.

The time barrier can usually be overcome by adding to activities that are already part of the patient's life, as described earlier, or by creating an exercise contract. A patient who feels that drastic action is needed to get active may find this method valuable. Other patients may find it too rigid. The patient creates the contract, which can either be with the counsellor or with him/herself, whichever is the most motivating for the patient. The contract should set out a certain day or days for exercise, a certain time on that day and a specific type of exercise that will be undertaken at that time. The contract can run for a mutually agreed time and revised as needed. A reward system can be built into successfully keeping the contract.

Not having anyone with whom to exercise can be very demotivating. Most people find it difficult not to go out for that swim when their best friend is standing at the door with towel and goggles all ready to go. Walking to the top of the hill to watch the sunset is far easier if you can chat all the way up with your next-door neighbour. Helping your patient to identify an 'exercise buddy' who will agree to work alongside them may be invaluable as a motivation tool, especially if the patient is a contemplator or preparer. A minority of people, however, much prefer to exercise alone.

The fears of discomfort and feelings of not being a sporty type are frequently generated by early bad experiences of physical education at school or subsequent weight gain, and will require great sensitivity from the exercise counsellor. The patient is likely to be in the precontemplator, contemplator or relapser group and may be fully aware that they should be more physically active for their own well-being, as well as to delay or prevent future diabetic complications. However, their deep dislike of physical activity makes it difficult for them even to think about starting. They may be resentful and unhappy about being in the exercise consultation room and are likely to have preconceived ideas about the unpleasantness of physical exercise. The counsellor needs to take a very supportive attitude, and to inform and educate about the benefits of even low intensity exercise for health. Working within the patient's current activity level is likely to yield the best results.

GOALS AND REWARDS

Goals and rewards are important for adults as well as children, and for patients in all categories of the Stages of Change model. The exercise counsellor has the task of finding out the appropriate goals and rewards for a specific individual: goals set too high will result in frustration; goals set too low may result in boredom. Patients in either of these states may drop out and stop being active. However, as in all other health care areas, it is best to work with the patient in setting the goals. Goal setting should include short-, medium- and long-term objectives and are best negotiated with the patient. Rewards are linked to the achieving of the goals and may be a prize or treat, or something more personal to the patient. Some patients may feel their reward is in performing in the annual show, having taken up tap dancing; others will aim for the London Marathon and find their reward is in competing successfully; yet others will be rewarded when they can manage to walk to the shops and back and still have energy to make the tea!

The moderate amount of physical activity associated with health benefits alone (outlined in Chapters 4 and 10) is achievable in most patients with a degree of encouragement and continued support. It is important that people with diabetes are able to identify types of exercise or physical activity that are both feasible and enjoyable. The ultimate aim of diabetes care is the longevity and quality of life enjoyed by each patient. Exercise and physical activity have an important part to play in realisation of these aims.

REFERENCES

1. Ruderman N, Horton E, Kemner F, Berger M. The Lost Symposium. *Diabetes Care* 1992; **15**: 959–960
2. American College of Sports Medicine. Position Statement: The Recommended Quantity and Quality of Exercise for Developing and Maintain-

ing Cardiorespiratory and Muscular Fitness in Healthy Adults. *Med Sci Sports Exerc* 1990; **25**: 265–274

3. Marsden, E. The role of exercise in the well-being of people with insulin dependent diabetes mellitus: perceptions of patients and health professionals. Doctoral thesis, Glasgow University, 1996
4. Morris JN, Everitt MG *et al.* Vigorous exercise in leisure time: protection against coronary heart disease. *Lancet* 1980; **2**: 1207–1210
5. Mutrie N, Loughlan C, Campbell M, Marsden E, McCarron T. The transtheoretical model applied to four Scottish populations. *J Sports Sci* 1997; **15**: 100
6. Canada Fitness Survey. Canadian Youth and Physical Activity. Ottowa, Canada Fitness Survey, 1983
7. Sports Council and Health Education Authority. *Allied Dunbar National Fitness Survey–Main Findings.* London, 1992
8. American Heart Association Scientific Council. Statement on Exercise. *Circulation* 1992; **86**: 340–344
9. Rippe JM, Ward A, Porcan JP, Freedson PS. Walking for health and fitness. *JAMA* 1988; **259**: 2720–2724
10. Leon AS, Connett J, Jacobs DR, Rauramaa R. Leisure time physical activity levels and risks of coronary heart disease and death: The Multiple Risk Factor Intervention Trial. *JAMA* 1987; **258**: 2388–2395
11. Slattery MC, Jacobs DR, Nichaman MZ. Leisure time physical activity, coronary heart disease and death: The US Railroad Study. *Circulation* 1989; **79**: 304–311
12. Centre for Disease Control and American College of Sports Medicine. Press Release. July 1993
13. Caspersen CJ, Powell KE, Christenson GM. Physical activity, exercise, and physical fitness. *Public Health Report* 1985; **100**: 125–131
14. Pate RR, Pratt M, Blair S *et al.* Physical activity and public health. *JAMA* 1995; **273**: 402–407
15. Berlin JA, Colditz GA. A meta-analysis of physical activity in the prevention of coronary heart disease. *Am J Epidemiol* 1990; **132**: 612–628
16. Blair SN, Kohl HW, Paffenberger RS, Clark DG, Cooper KH, Gibbons LW. Physical fitness and all-cause mortality. *JAMA* 1989; **262**: 2395–2401
17. Blair SN, Kohl HW, Gordon NF, Paffenberger RS. How much physical activity is good for health? *Ann Rev Publ Health* 1992; **13**: 99–126
18. Borg GA, Psychological bases of perceived exertion. *Med Sci Sports and Exer* 1982; **14**: 377–387
19. Wimbush E. A moderate approach to promoting physical activity: the evidence and implications. *Health Educ J* 1994; **53**: 322–336
20. Berg K. *Diabetic's guide to health and fitness.* Champaign, IL: Human Kinetics, 1986

21. Sallis J, Hovell M. Determinants of exercise behaviour. *Exer Sports Sci Rev* 1990; **18**: 307–330

22. Prochaska JO, DiClemente CC. Transtheoretical therapy: towards a more integrative model of change. *Psychother Theory, Res Pract* 1982; **20**: 161–173

23. Prochaska JO, Marcus B. The transtheoretical model: applications to exercise. In: Dishman RK (ed.) *Advances in Exercise Adherence*. Champaign, IL: Human Kinetics, 1995

24. DiClemente CC, Prochaska JO. Self change and therapy change of smoking behaviour: a comparison of process of cessation and maintenance. *Addict Behav* 1982; **7**: 133–142

25. Marcus B, Selby V, Niaura R, Rossi J. Self-efficacy and the stages of exercise behavior change. *Res Quart Exerc Sport* 1992; **63**: 50–66

26. Marcus BH, Banspach SW, Lefebvre RC *et al.* Using stages of changes model to increase the adoption of physical activity among community participants. *Am J Health Promotion* 1992; **6**: 424–429

27. Oldridge NB. Compliance and exercise in primary and secondary prevention of coronary heart disease: a review. *Prevent Med* 1982; **11**: 56–70

28. Morris JN. Exercise in the prevention of coronary heart disease: today's best buy in public health. *Med Sci Sport Exerc* 1993; 807–813

29. Health Education Authority. *Promoting physical activity in primary health care*. London: HEA, 1996

30. Biddle S, Mutrie N. Exercise adoption and maintenance. In: *Psychology of physical activity and exercise*. London: Springer Verlag, 1991, pp. 27–61

31. Ashford B, Biddle S. Participation in community sports centres: motives and predictors of enjoyment. Paper presented to the British Association of Sports Science Conference, Cardiff, 1990

32. Paffenbarger RS, Hyde RT, Wing RL. Physical activity and physical fitness as determinants of health and longevity. In: Bouchard C, Shephard RJ, Stephens T, Sutton JR, Mcpherson BD (eds). *Exercise fitness and Health: A consensus of current knowledge*. Champaign, IL: Human Kinetics, 1990, pp. 33–48

33. Pender NJ, Pender AR. Attitudes, subjective norms and intentions to engage in health research. *Nurs Res* 1986; **35**: 15–18

34. Rhodes E, Dunwoody D. Physiological and attitudinal changes in those involved in an employee fitness program. *Can J Public Health* 1980; **71**: 331–336

35. Iverson DC, Fielding JE, Crow RS, Christenson GM. The promotion of physical activity in the United States' population: the status of programmes in medical, worksite, community and school settings. *Public Health Rep* 1985; **100**: 212–224

36. Shephard R. Motivation: the key to fitness compliance. *Phys Sports Med* 1985; **13:** 88–101
37. Loughlan C, Mutrie N. An evaluation of the effectiveness of three interventions in promoting physical activity in a sedentary population. *Health Educ J* 1997; **56:** 154–165

APPENDIX 1

The calf stretch (Figure 9.3): Face a wall and place both hands at shoulder height on the wall. Both feet are pointing towards the wall. Take the left foot back 2–3 feet, keeping the heel flat on the floor. Lean gently forward until the stretch can be felt in the left calf muscle. Hold the position when a full stretch is achieved. Slowly change legs and repeat.

Quadriceps stretch (Figure 9.4): Standing sideways to the wall and using nearest hand to balance, use the outside hand to bring the outside foot backwards towards the small of the back. Keep knees fairly close together. To reach full stretch, it may be necessary to gently push hips forwards. Hold for 15–30 seconds then turn to stand other side to the wall. Slowly stretch the other leg.

Hamstring stretch (Figure 9.5): Lying on the floor with the left knee bent, slowly bring the other straightened leg towards the chest. Try to relax the right hamstring as it is being stretched. Repeat with the other leg.

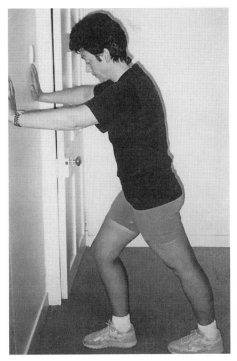

Figure 9.3. Calf stretch

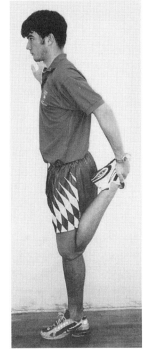

Figure 9.4. Quadriceps stretch

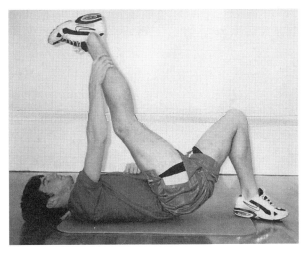

Figure 9.5. Hamstring stretch

Groin stretch (Figure 9.6): Sitting with the feet apart and backs of legs on the ground, gradually walk fingers forward until a full stretch in the groin is felt. Hold. This position also stretches the back and the shoulders.

Gluteus maximus stretch (Figure 9.7): Lying on the floor with the left knee bent, bring the outside of the right foot to rest on top of the left knee. Slowly lift the left foot from the ground until a stretch can be felt in the right gluteus maximus. Hold for 15-30 seconds before changing legs.

Stretch for the small of the back (Figure 9.8): Lying with both knees pulled up to the chest, grasp the knees with both arms and slowly bring up the forehead towards the knees. Hold.

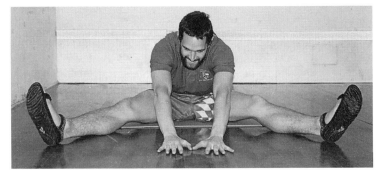

Figure 9.6. Groin stretch

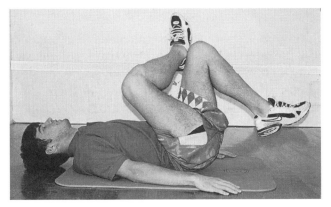

Figure 9.7. Gluteus maximus stretch

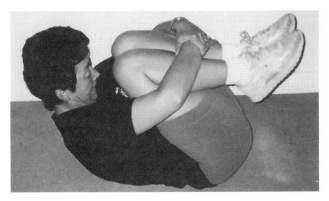

Figure 9.8. Small of the back stretch

Side stretch (Figure 9.9): Standing with feet 2-3 feet apart, bend to the left and allow the left hand to support the trunk weight by leaning on the left hip or thigh. Stretch the right arm over the top. Return to the upright position after 15 seconds and repeat to the right. Try not to allow the trunk to fall forwards or backwards.

Chest and shoulder stretch (Figure 9.10): Join hands and lift them both behind the back towards shoulder height. Hold and relax.

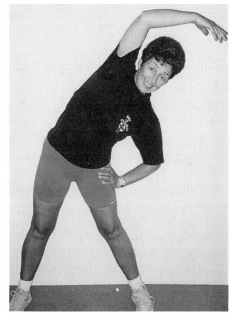

Figure 9.9. Side stretch

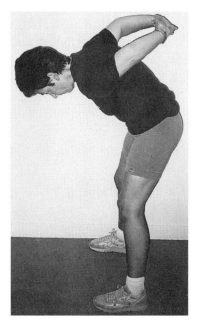

Figure 9.10. Chest and shoulder stretch

Shoulder stretch (Figure 9.11): Lift the right arm above the head, bend at the elbow and drop the right hand behind the shoulder. Use the other hand to grasp the right elbow and ease it gently backwards to reach full stretch. Hold for 15-30 seconds before changing arms.

Full body stretch (Figure 9.12): With feet comfortably apart, link fingers together and turn the palms upwards. Lift hands above the head so that palms are facing towards the roof. Push hands away from body centre to achieve a full body stretch. This stretch can also be performed lying on the floor with toes also fully stretched.

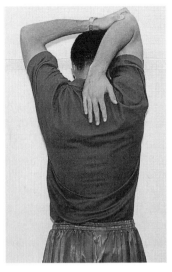

Figure 9.11. Shoulder Stretch

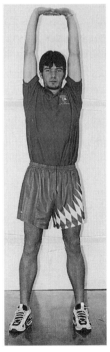

Figure 9.12. Full body stretch

APPENDIX 2

Heel raises (calves) (Figure 9.13): Facing a wall, rest both hands on the wall at shoulder level for balance. Start with the feet flat on the floor, then raise heels as high as possible whilst keeping the balls of the feet on the floor.

Half squats (quadriceps, glutei, hamstrings) (Figure 9.14): With feet 2–3 feet apart, bend and then straighten knees, keeping back straight. Knees should be bent only far enough to allow thighs to be parallel with floor.

Trunk curl (rectus abdominis, internal and external oblique) (Figure 9.15): Lying comfortably on the back with both knees bent, first tuck the chin to the chest then flex the spine so that consecutive vertebrae are raised from the ground. The exercise is complete when the trunk is about 30° to the floor.

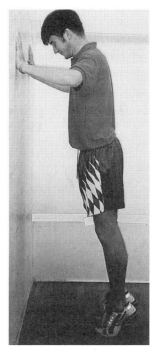

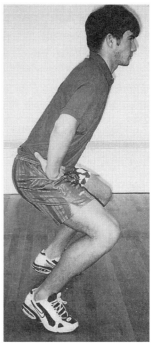

Figure 9.13.   Heel raises

Figure 9.14.   Half squat

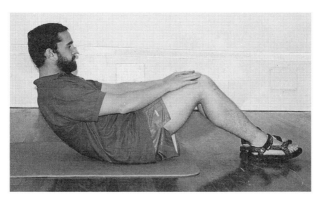

Figure 9.15.   Trunk curl

Back raises (latissimus dorsi, trapezius, infraspinatus and teres major and minor) (Figure 9.16): Lying face down with hands under the chin and elbows flexed, use the back muscles to raise the upper part of the body slowly from the ground. Hips and lower part of body remain on the floor.

Press ups (pectorals, triceps, deltoids) (Figure 9.17): This exercise may be performed against the wall, from the knees and hands or from the toes and hands. Hands are placed below the shoulders and elbows are straightened and bent. To avoid undue strain on the lower back, it is best to keep the hips slightly bent.

Rowing pull (biceps, triceps, latissimus dorsi, teres major and minor, subscapularis, supraspinatus, infraspinatus, rhomboids) (Figure 9.18): Bending at the knees and using a chair or bench on which to lean, grasp a small weight in one hand and pull it towards the chest. Return the weight to brush the floor before lifting again. Change arms for the next set.

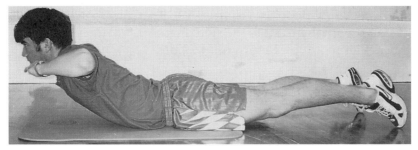

Figure 9.16. Back raises

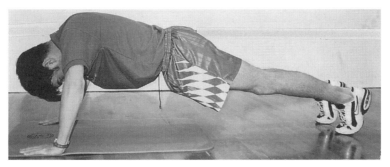

Figure 9.17. Press ups

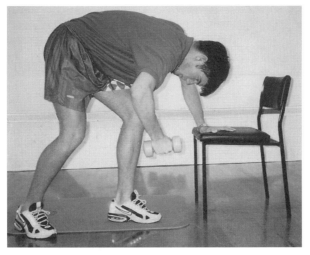

Figure 9.18. Rowing pull

Pec-dec (pectorals, deltoids) (Figure 9.19): Keeping elbows at shoulder height, start with them out to the side (Figure 9.19a) then bring elbows together (Figure 9.19b). Return out to sides.

The good exercise or physical exercise programme ends with another period of flexibility and stretching.

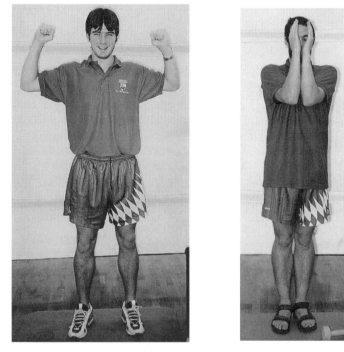

(a)   (b)

Figure 9.19.   Pec-dec

10

The Role of the Diabetes Team in Promoting Physical Activity

BILL BURR AND DINESH NAGI

Pinderfields Hospital, Wakefield, UK

INTRODUCTION

In people with type 1 diabetes, there are no proven benefits of exercise in terms of improved glycaemic control. The importance of physical activity and sport in these people is related largely to the way that it can prove to be a barrier, especially in the young, which may prevent them from taking part in activities they would otherwise enjoy. It is hoped that the advice contained in earlier chapters (2, 5, 7 and 8) may help to avoid this unfortunate development. Those with type 1 diabetes may still share in the general health benefits which accrue to those taking regular exercise, and it is worth remembering that inactive people who do *not* have diabetes have twice the risk of premature death and serious illness as those who keep active[1]. In addition, sedentary living is now recognised to be the fourth primary risk factor for coronary heart disease behind hypertension, hyper-cholesterolaemia, and smoking[2,3]. People with type 1 diabetes have an increased risk of coronary artery disease, and those who keep active should expect to enjoy benefits in terms of reduced risk of cardio-vascular disease, as well as the improved exercise capacity and psychological well-being associated with physical activity[4].

Exercise and Sport in Diabetes. Edited by Bill Burr and Dinesh Nagi.
© 1999 John Wiley & Sons Ltd.

The role of the diabetes team in relation to type 1 diabetes involves having the knowledge, interest, time and educational materials to help patients to take part safely in their chosen sport.

In contrast, the health benefits of regular physical activity in type 2 diabetes have been clearly established, are evidence-based[5], and were reviewed in detail in Chapter 4. They include improved glycaemic control, reduced cardiovascular risks, reduced adiposity, increased physical fitness, and improved psychological well-being. It follows that increased physical activity is a fundamental part of the treatment package for type 2 diabetes, and the diabetes team has a clear requirement to promote and encourage this.

Unfortunately, our success in achieving the lifestyle alterations necessary for good control in type 2 patients has been limited. The results of the recently published UK Prospective Diabetes Study confirm this in terms of weight control[6]. The conventionally treated group increased weight by approximately 5 kg during median follow-up of 10 years, and the intensively treated group increased weight by about 10 kg, which is extremely disappointing given the importance of weight loss for successful management of the condition. There is no reason to believe that our success in promoting increased physical activity is any better.

Patients are either not receiving the message about the importance of lifestyle changes or are unable to act upon the advice given. Lifestyle changes are never easy to achieve, but we must ask ourselves why patients are not managing to do what is required.

- Is it due to a failure to inform patients about the benefits of regular physical exercise?
- Is it due to failure of the patients to break down the barriers to physical activity in spite of adequate knowledge about the need to be more active?
- Is it due to a general lack of social and emotional support for these patients to help them to achieve and sustain an increase in physical activity?

It is likely that all these factors combine to varying degrees in different patients. Strategies for dealing with these problems are dealt with later, but at this point it is relevant to consider whether the topic of physical activity is routinely being addressed in most diabetic clinics.

EDUCATING THE DIABETES TEAM

There is a need for all health professionals dealing with type 2 diabetes to understand the crucial role of increasing physical activity in treating the disease. We recently surveyed such professionals working in the UK. Most were aware of the benefits of physical activity, but spent very little time on physical activity assessment and education. A majority felt that the advice currently being offered is inadequate, unlikely to lead to lifestyle changes, and in need of improvement. The findings suggested that there is an awareness of the increasing importance of exercise in diabetes management, but that there may be a problem of identifying time, staff and facilities to deal properly with the subject (unpublished observations).

The make-up of diabetes teams has been mainly influenced by the care requirements of patients with type 1 diabetes and its complications. This accounts for the inclusion of doctors, dietitians, specialist nurses and podiatrists in most diabetes teams, sometimes with the addition of a psychologist. The care requirements of people with type 2 diabetes have usually had to be fitted into a pattern of care developed for insulin-treated patients. Unlike type 1 disease, type 2 diabetes is a lifestyle disease, and successful treatment requires adjustments of diet, weight and physical activity. Patients have to be persuaded and motivated to make these changes and to sustain them over many years, even though they may have few, if any, symptoms. This requires a high standard of communication and educational skills as well as an ability to motivate.

These attributes are not necessarily the same as those possessed by diabetologists, nurse specialists or dietitians, and this may partly explain our limited success in treating type 2 diabetes. It may be that members of the primary care team are better equipped to take on this role, although without appropriate education they may not appreciate the crucial importance of lifestyle changes. They should not, for instance, be too ready to introduce drug therapies such as sulphonylureas and insulin, which can, by encouraging weight gain, make the metabolic syndrome even more difficult to treat.

EXERCISE THERAPIST AS PART OF THE TEAM?

As we realise that the fundamental deficiency state in type 2 diabetes is not one of beta cell secretion but of physical activity, then the need for a member of the diabetes team to have expert knowledge of this area becomes obvious. Such a person may have enthusiasm and knowledge about the benefits of physical activity. Unfortunately, their effectiveness is likely to be limited by other commitments and a person with primary expertise in exercise, who understands the importance of physical activity in diabetes, such as a hospital or community-based physiotherapist, might have a role in this area.

The exercise therapist would be able to work with other members of the diabetes team to produce physical activity programmes appropriate for a patient's state of health. He or she should also be able to lead group activity programmes—which seem to be particularly successful with female patients—and could supervise exercise sessions in a gym, physiotherapy department or diabetes centre; such sessions at the beginning of a weight loss programme have been shown to improve success rates[7]. Group sessions help to demonstrate to people the kind of activities and aerobic exercises they can perform safely, and give an opportunity for a person to meet others who are in a similar situation.

In a broader context, the exercise therapist should be able to educate other groups dealing with diabetes care about the most effective ways of motivating and guiding patients to take more exercise.

Whether a specialist exercise therapist should be based in primary or secondary care should not be a critical issue. Wherever they are based, it is important that there should be close working relationships with both primary and secondary care in order to promote educational activity.

ASSESSMENT OF PATIENTS

Every patient needs full evaluation before commencing exercise. This will include a medical examination as well as an assessment of current levels of physical activity, and attitudes to exercise.

The medical (generally done by a physician) examination should include:

1. Medical history. Any history of:
   - heart disease, angina, previous coronary thrombosis or coronary artery bypass
   - peripheral vascular disease
   - stroke or transient ischaemic attack
   - hypertension
   - diabetic complications, such as retinopathy, neuropathy or nephropathy
2. Social history:
   - occupation
   - history of smoking and alcohol intake
3. Physical examination and investigations:
   - body mass index
   - pulse, blood pressure, peripheral pulses
   - foot examination
   - retinopathy screen
   - biochemical investigations or ECG if indicated

After the medical evaluation, when any barriers to physical activity related to diabetes or other medical conditions have been identified, the patient ideally should meet the team member responsible for exercise promotion, who will assess and advise on the following:

- Current physical activity
- Knowledge about benefits/risks of exercise
- Attitudes and barriers to taking exercise
- Psychosocial and economic factors
- Tips for safe activities
- Self-monitoring through exercise diaries
- Goal setting—frequency, type, duration of physical activity. Weight targets for obese
- Frequency of contact, supervision (for motivation and confidence building)

THE EXERCISE PRESCRIPTION

For many people with diabetes, especially those with type 2 disease and those starting to exercise, a prescription for even moderate exercise would be impossible. It is important to get over the message that every little helps. The daily exercise target can be built up in small parcels of activity, so it is vital to stress the importance of seemingly trivial activities such as avoiding the use of lifts and escalators, parking a little further from the supermarket, getting off at a bus stop which is not the nearest etc. The exercise prescription for health improvement has already been stated in earlier chapters, but can be summarised as being equivalent to 30 minutes of moderate physical exertion (such as very brisk (4 mph) walking), on five or six days a week. If the exertion is of lesser or greater intensity, then it should be continued for a shorter or longer periods, as suggested in Table 10.1. General advice about the safety of exercise, and the necessary precautions to avoid disturbances of diabetic control, have been

Table 10.1. The exercise prescription: recommended examples of moderate physical activity

30 minutes
- Walking very briskly on flat (2 miles, 4 mph), or carrying 25-lb load at 3 mph
- Gardening—weeding, mowing lawn (power mower), raking lawn
- Home—sweeping up, washing and waxing car, painting/plastering, washing windows
- Cycling leisurely (10 mph—5 miles in 30 min)
- Dancing—ballroom
- Golf—using trolley for clubs
- Volleyball
- Badminton—doubles
- Horse riding

20 minutes
- Walking upstairs, backpacking, mountain walking
- Running (5 mph)
- Swimming (slow crawl, 50 yards/min)
- Mowing lawn (hand mower)
- Tennis (singles)
- Basketball
- Cycling moderate effort (12–14 mph)

Activities to be performed ideally 5–6 times per week

Adapted from Ainsworth *et al.*[14]

given in previous chapters (2, 4, 7). The watchword for those starting to exercise is to *start low and go slow*—begin with small increases compared to current activity and build up gradually. Report any untoward symptoms to medical advisers.

We feel that most patients with diabetes can increase their physical activity levels, with the type of activity being determined by an individual's personal preference, current lifestyle, and any physical limitations/complications which may exist. The exercise prescription needs to be individualised and to achieve this a detailed knowledge of a person's diabetes, lifestyle, and beliefs about physical activity is very important. This enables the members of the diabetes team, in collaboration with the patient and his/her family, to discuss and formulate a structured programme of physical activity to optimise the health gains of exercise with minimal risk.

PATIENT EDUCATION

Education regarding the benefits of physical activity should ideally be introduced at the time of initial diagnosis when the motivation for behaviour change is at its highest. Great care needs to be taken to give special emphasis to the exercise prescription, which might otherwise be lost among more immediate problems such as diet and blood testing. In this context, it is helpful that adopting physical activity is a positive health behaviour—in contrast to many negative associations that go with the diagnosis of diabetes, such as restrictions on favourite foods, alcohol and smoking.

Most diabetes clinics do not at present allocate a specific place for education about physical activity in their programmes for people with type 2 diabetes. We have made preliminary observations, which suggest that allocating a small amount of time for focussed advice about physical activity can significantly increase the levels of self-reported activity during the next 6 months[8].

There are currently very few resource materials available to diabetes teams to assist them in their efforts to promote physical activity in patients, particularly those with type 2 disease. In the UK, the Health Education Council produces materials for exercise promotion for use by community and health professionals, but these are not specifically targeted to the problems of people with diabetes[9]. In promoting exercise and managing weight loss, graphs may be useful which show, for instance, the increased longevity associated with weight loss in newly diagnosed type 2 patients (Figure 10.1).

Other information, which confirms the benefits of weight loss in terms of reduced risk of diabetes, improved diabetes control, lower blood pressure and lipid levels, and improved survival (Table 10.2) may be useful for the education of health professionals and, with suitable adaptation, for education of patients. Material produced primarily to highlight the benefits of weight loss may be used while discussing the advantages of physical activity, since increased activity has been shown to maintain weight loss. We need a better selection of eye-catching and persuasive material to highlight the benefits of physical activity.

MOTIVATING PATIENTS AND CHANGING BEHAVIOUR

When attempting to motivate patients towards becoming more active, it is worth noting that the very word 'exercise' has strong negative associations for the type of person we are usually trying to encourage.

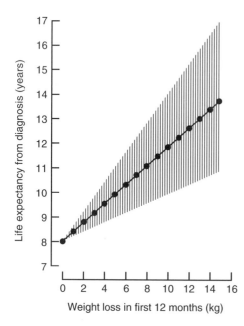

Figure 10.1. Life expectancy in patients with type 2 diabetes (BMI> 26 kg/m^2) in relation to weight loss in the first year of treatment. The shaded area represents the 95% confidence intervals. Adapted from Lean *et al.*,[15] by permission

Table 10.2. Potential health benefits of 10 kg weight loss in a patient weighing 100 kg

---

Mortality:
- 20–25% fall in total mortality
- 30–40% fall in diabetes-related deaths
- 40–50% fall in obesity-related cancer deaths

Blood pressure:
- Fall of approx 10 mmHg in systolic/diastolic

Diabetes:
- > 50% reduction in risk of developing diabetes
- 30–50% fall in fasting glucose
- 15% fall in HbAlc

Lipids:
- 10% fall in total cholesterol
- 15% fall in LDL cholesterol
- 30% fall in triglycerides
- 8% increase in HDL cholesterol

Adapted from Jung RT, *Br Med Bull* 1997; **53:** 307–321 by permission

In many people's minds it is linked to visions of youth and athletic endeavour, and it is important that we take care not to foster this notion by our choice of words. For this reason we deliberately choose to talk about 'physical activity', rather than 'exercise' or 'sport'.

In the previous chapter the 'Stages of Change' model was detailed as an approach to achieving lifestyle alterations. Briefly, according to this model, it is necessary to establish the patient's attitude to increasing physical activity before deciding on the approach to take. Some will have given the idea no thought at all, consider it to be a waste of time or unimportant, and have no intention of starting to exercise (pre-contemplators). Others may have accepted that they should be taking more exercise, but will have not yet made any changes (contemplators), while some will actually be trying to do more (action), and yet others may have tried and failed (relapse). Finally, there will be some who have been successful in making change but need support to sustain this change. Having established where the patient lies on the spectrum of stages of change, it is possible to derive appropriate strategies to help them to move from one stage to another, ensuring that interventions are matched to the patient's state of mind, and therefore most likely to meet with success.

Patients are likely to need a great deal of encouragement and support, especially in the early stages when they are at the stage of 'action' or are ready for action. Encouragement may take the form of providing information, recounting difficulties encountered by others, or lending a sympathetic ear to problems which the patient may be having. Even the most committed individuals who exercise on a regular basis need some recognition and support from time to time.

BARRIERS TO PHYSICAL ACTIVITY

These may be physical or psychological. The physical are probably more easy to recognise, and have to be allowed for in developing a safe exercise plan. However, it is important also to keep in mind the various psychological factors which can lead to negative attitudes and experiences which are likely to prevent patients from exercising:

- 'Not being a sporty type' is the most common reason given by middle-aged or older people for not taking exercise[10]. It must be linked to a lack of knowledge about the relatively low levels of physical activity required in order to benefit health, and should therefore be relatively easy to overcome during initial education (see Table 10.1).
- Embarrassment about physique is a major problem in dealing with the obese type 2 patient, especially females. It can be a complete bar to them taking part in activities such as swimming, which in other respects is an ideal activity for these patients. It may sometimes be dealt with successfully in group activities, where others have the same problems, so that group aerobic or swimming sessions can help to break down initial embarrassment. Educational materials which feature overweight people in a favourable manner can also be very helpful in boosting confidence to allow such patients to start exercising.
- Self-confidence. Obese and inactive people are likely to have low levels of self-esteem, and the diagnosis of diabetes is probably going to reduce this still further. These people are very likely to

have negative attitudes to their body image, and to the idea of taking exercise. The fact that control of diabetes requires that the issues of weight and inactivity are confronted is almost certainly going to provoke even more negative responses. The health professional needs to be sensitive to the vulnerable state of the newly-diagnosed type 2 patient. Goals in relation to both exercise and diet need to be realistic, to ensure that the patient is capable of achieving them. In this way confidence can progressively be built up as activity increases. At the same time, the professional needs to be generous with praise to promote the confidence-building exercise.

GOAL SETTING

It has been suggested that the use of 'decision balance sheets' (Table 10.3), may increase commitment for a behaviour change, particularly at the outset[11]. This would include setting an initial feasible and easily achievable target with high likelihood of success. For example, this might involve a decision (as illustrated) to walk on three days a week. Potential benefits and negatives are listed and given values to reflect their relative importance to the patient. Over a period of time the patient can work with the health professional in charge of exercise promotion to review and change targets, and to maximise benefits and reduce the impact of negative factors[12]. This goal-setting exercise is a useful way of establishing new exercise habits, and this can be reinforced if the patient also keeps an activity record that can be used to build on successes and to help formulate new targets. The initial aim is to build up the frequency of exercise, followed by exercise duration and then intensity.

THE COMMUNITY AND NATIONAL CONTEXT

We live in a society that has witnessed the development of a lifestyle whereby almost 40% of 55–74-year-old people indulge in no measurable physical activity[10]. There is an urgent need to develop local and national schemes to promote physical activity as a means of preventing cardiovascular disease as well as type 2 diabetes. Attempts to promote physical activity in the UK have met with little success to

Table 10.3. Exercise decision balance sheet

<table>
<tr><td colspan="4" style="text-align:center">Walking back to health:
Your personal decision balance sheet</td></tr>
<tr><td colspan="4">Target behaviour:
Taking three 30-minute lunchtime walks on Monday, Wednesday and Friday this week.</td></tr>
<tr><td>Reasons for exercising*</td><td>Impact</td><td>Reasons against exercising*</td><td>Impact</td></tr>
<tr><td>I know it will make me feel better</td><td>☐</td><td>I can't seem to find the time</td><td>☐</td></tr>
<tr><td>It will help me manage my weight</td><td>☐</td><td>I don't really know what I have to do</td><td>☐</td></tr>
<tr><td>I enjoy getting out of the house</td><td>☐</td><td>I feel embarrassed about exercise</td><td>☐</td></tr>
<tr><td>It makes me feel fitter and in control</td><td>☐</td><td>I feel guilty about taking the time</td><td>☐</td></tr>
<tr><td>It is something positive I can do</td><td>☐</td><td>I find it painful</td><td>☐</td></tr>
<tr><td>I want to show others that I can do it</td><td>☐</td><td>There is nowhere safe to exercise</td><td>☐</td></tr>
<tr><td>Other ....</td><td>☐</td><td>Other ....</td><td>☐</td></tr>
<tr><td>Other ....</td><td>☐</td><td>Other ....</td><td>☐</td></tr>
<tr><td>Total positive impact</td><td>☐</td><td>Total negative impact</td><td>☐</td></tr>
<tr><td colspan="4">Strategies for improvement
• Add in more positive reasons or make existing ones more powerful— e.g. I enjoy walking as it makes me spend time with my friends
• Eliminate or reduce the reasons against—I have talked about walking for health with my family and they want to help me find some personal time. I now feel supported and less guilty</td></tr>
<tr><td colspan="4">*Patients should be encouraged to generate their own lists of positive and negative factors</td></tr>
</table>

Adapted from reference 12, by permission

date. A successful national campaign to increase physical activity would help the targeted efforts of diabetes teams in encouraging those with established diabetes to increase their activity levels. In the meantime, diabetes teams should exploit every opportunity to publicise the health risks of obesity and inactivity.

In summary, we feel that;

1. All subjects with type 2 diabetes should be assessed for their leisure time and occupational activity.
2. They should be screened for complications of diabetes before starting a formal exercise programme.
3. Those who currently take little or no exercise but are ready for action should be given individualised advice to encourage increased activity.
4. All patients with type 2 diabetes should have education regarding exercise, and this should form an essential part of ongoing education.
5. Diabetes teams should take a lead role in developing information leaflets and highlighting the health benefits of exercise.

The following case histories illustrate some of the benefits of increased physical activity in patients with type 2 diabetes. We have included them in the hope that this will encourage colleagues to adopt similar strategies for dealing with the lifestyle problems of such patients.

CASE HISTORY 1

A 46-year-old man was diagnosed as having type 2 diabetes at the age of 31 and was followed up at another hospital. He was seen at the Edna Coates Diabetes Centre in August 1995. He had no symptoms of hyperglycaemia and had noticed that his blood sugars at home had been running 'high'. He was a non-smoker and drank 16 units of alcohol a week. His medication was metformin 850 mg tds and glibenclamide 5 mg bd. His weight was 93.1 kg, BMI 27, blood pressure 131/84 mmHg, HbA1c 10.6% (3.1–5.0).

The patient was commenced on insulin treatment, and in July 1996 he weighed 104.6 kg, his HbA1c was 5.7%, and he was taking 45 units of Humulin I twice daily. He had gained 11.6 kg, although there had also been a dramatic improvement in his diabetic control. However, in

November 1996, his control had slipped back: HbA1c of 7.3% and weight 106 kg. As he was concerned about weight gain, and his diabetic control had worsened, he was advised to take up regular physical activity. Six months later, he had managed to reduce his insulin by a total of 20 units/day and his HbA1c had improved to 5.8%. He had converted his garage into a mini gym and exercised 60 min/day 3–4 days/week. In addition to reducing his total dose of insulin by about 25%, his diabetic control had improved. The patient felt 'excellent' and physically fit, with improved quality of life.

CASE HISTORY 2

A 53-year-old woman was found to have type 2 diabetes in May 1991, and was markedly symptomatic. She weighed 134 kg (BMI 50.3), and was commenced on diet and metformin 500 mg tds. In Jan 1992, she weighed 125 kg, had no glycosuria and was lost to follow up (she was worried that she had not lost enough weight and would be 'told off'). She was seen again at the diabetes centre in June 1997, because she was again symptomatic, and surprisingly weighed 99 kg, BMI 37, HbA1c 8.8%. In August 1997 she weighed 93.7 kg and was taking metformin 850 mg tds. In addition, she had started floor exercises, 20 minutes daily, walked for 90 min most days of the week, and took stairs to her office (situated on the 11th floor). She had instituted a strict programme of diet and exercise and in 12 months had lost nearly 21 kg, while her glycaemic control improved slightly, with HbA1c of 8.3%.

There are two messages from this case. First, she had done well first time around, having lost about 6% of total body weight, and should have been congratulated on her achievements. Secondly, building a programme of exercise that fits into one's lifestyle is likely to be sustained in the long run.

CASE HISTORY 3

A 49-year-old male non-obese subject with type 2 diabetes presented in October 1995 with osmotic symptoms, and was commenced on treatment with diet and gliclazide 80 mg once daily. His HbA1c was 9.9%, and gliclazide was increased to 80 mg twice daily. In April 1996, he was seen at the diabetes centre and had a BMI of 25, 5% glycosuria and HbA1c of 7.4%. Metformin was added at 500 mg tds. In July 1996, his glycaemic control had deteriorated further and HbA1c had risen to 9.0%. He was advised to take regular physical activity, and 6 months later had a HbA1c of 6.8%. He was now walking 30 min during his lunch break and 60 min in the evening.

CONCLUSIONS

There is good evidence that increased physical activity leads to a number of health benefits, which are particularly important in the treatment and prevention of type 2 diabetes. Diabetes teams need to provide full information about the role of inactivity in the causation of type 2 diabetes, and the fact that successful treatment requires an increase in physical activity. They also need to be able to motivate patients to be more active, and to provide long-term support to maintain behaviour change[11]. Diabetes teams need to give exercise promotion at least equal importance to advice concerning diet and disease monitoring; this is likely to require extra resources as well as a great deal of commitment from members of the team. Whatever programmes we design and implement to promote physical activity, will have to be evaluated to determine their cost effectiveness in the overall management of type 2 diabetes[13].

REFERENCES

1. Killoran AJ, Fentem P, Casperson C, eds. *Moving On: International Perspectives on Promoting Physical Activity.* London: Health Education Authority, 1994
2. Powell KE, Thompson PD, Casperson CJ, Ford ES. Physical activity and the incidence of coronary heart disease. *Annu Rev Public Health* 1987; **8:** 253–287
3. Berlin JA, Colditz GA. A meta-analysis of physical activity in the prevention of coronary heart disease. *Am J Epidemiol* 1990; **132:** 612–628
4. Blair SN, Hardman A. Special issue: Physical activity, health and well-being—an international consensus conference. *Res Q Exerc Sport* 1995; **66** (4)
5. American Diabetes Association: Exercise and NIDDM (Technical Review). *Diabetes Care* 1990; **13:** 785–789

6. United Kingdom Prospective Diabetes Study Group. UK prospective diabetes study 33: intensive blood glucose control with sulphonylureas or insulin compared with conventional treatment and risk of complications in patients with type 2 diabetes. *Lancet* 1998; **352:** 837–853

7. Craighead LW, Blum MD. Supervised exercise in behavioural treatment for moderate obesity. *Behav Ther* 1989; **20:** 49–59

8. Berlanga F, Wareham N, Burr WA, Nagi DK. Does a 'focused' advice to increase physical activity work in patients with newly diagnosed type 2 diabetes? *Diabetic Med* 1998; (Suppl. 1): S24

9. Health Education Authority. *A Guide to Physical Activity Promotion in Primary Care in England*. London: Health Education Authority, 1996

10. Health Education Authority and Sports Council. *Allied Dunbar National Fitness Survey: Main Findings*. London: Health Education Authority, 1992

11. Wankel LM. Decision-making and social support strategies for increasing exercise involvement. *J Cardiac Rehabil* 1984; **4:** 124–135

12. Fox KR. Promoting physical activity in people with diabetes. *Practical Diabetes International* 1998; **15:** 146–150

13. Graber Al, Christman BG, Alogna MT, Davidson JK. Evaluation of diabetes patient education programme. *Diabetes* 1977; **26:** 61–64

14. Ainsworth BE, Haskell WL, Leon AS *et al.* Compendium of physical activities: classification of energy costs of human activities. *Med Sci Sports Exerc* 1993; **25:** 71–80

15. Lean ME, Powrie JK, Anderson AS, Garthwaite PH. Obesity, weight loss and prognosis in type 2 diabetes. *Diabetic Med* 1990; **7:** 228–233

Index

Index compiled by Liza Weinkove